THE OXYGEN MASK MINDSET

Reclaiming Your Energy in a World that Glorifies Exhaustion

Calissa Ngozi

✿ LUCKY BOOK PUBLISHING

To request permissions, contact the publisher at hello@luckybookpublishing.com.

Paperback ISBN: 978-1-997775-01-0
Hardcover ISBN: 978-1-997775-00-3
E-book ISBN: 978-1-998287-99-4

First edition, August 2025

In The Oxygen Mask Mindset, Calissa Ngozi offers the loving nudge we need to see self-care for what it truly is: self-preservation.

-Tara Slone, Sirius XM Host
and Juno Award Nominee

Dedication & Heart Acknowledgments

To my twins, Hunter and Sawyer

You are my heart song. You are the reason I breathe deeper, dream bigger, and keep showing up. You gave me purpose before I fully knew my own. Everything I do is to model a world where rest, joy, and mental wellness are not luxuries but birthrights.

To my parents, John and Wendy

Thank you for choosing me. For loving me as your own, giving me the gift of faith and a relationship with God, and shaping the foundation of who I am. You gave me a chance at life, and I'm building something beautiful with it.

To my ex-husband, Daniel

Thank you for being a damn good co-parent. Your presence and flexibility allows me to pour into our children and pour into my purpose. That balance is rare, and I don't take it for granted.

To Dan and Rina from SpeakerSlam

You were the launchpad. You cracked me open and handed me the mic. Because of you, my voice became more than a whisper-it became a calling. Thank you for believing in me before the world caught up.

To my dear friend and mentor, Declan

You saw the greatness in me when all I saw was survival. Thank you for holding up the mirror when I needed to remember who the hell I am.

To my sister and soul anchor, Trissy

You are my soft place. The one who holds space for me exactly how I need. Your presence is a healing salve I never have to earn. I love you more than words know how to say. Special shout out to her husband, my "Brother-In-Love" Furman, for always being there for anything I need, and constantly encouraging my relationship with my sister.

To my cousin, Michelle

My lifelong cheerleader. My hype woman. My steady support. You've always made me feel seen, and that's a gift I'll never stop being grateful for.

To Myself

Thank you for choosing you. For doing the messy, terrifying, powerful work of healing. For turning your pain into purpose. For investing in your story. For speaking the truth even when your voice shook. You didn't write this book to become someone new. You wrote it to come home to yourself.

And finally to you, the reader

Thank you for trusting me with your time, your heart, your exhaustion, and your hope. Thank you for indulging my sass, my soul, and my story. Most of all, thank you for choosing you. This book isn't just mine anymore—it's ours.

Let's breathe.

Let's rise.

Let's **reclaim it all**.

MY GIFT TO YOU

I am so glad you're here!

As my Gift to you, get FREE Access to
The Oxygen Mask Mindset bonus content
by scanning the QR Code below or visiting

www.CalissaNgozi.com/books

My Dream

Dear Reader,

Burnout is real. Full Stop. It's not about laziness or a lack of grit and perseverance. It is about pressure that piles up until your brain and body can't handle it any longer.

If this book is in your hands, you might be running on fumes. Bone-deep, soul-deep fatigue. I am not just talking about physically, but emotionally, mentally, and spiritually. Maybe you're juggling boardroom deadlines or bedtime stories or both, and everything feels overwhelming.

My dream for this book is simple. I want it to land in every pair of hands, from normal folks to corporate climbers, from worn-out moms to high-level execs. I want it to be seen as a friend on the journey, not a trophy at the finish line. Come back to these pages when you need to, not just one and done.

This book isn't a one-time pep talk. It's a practice. You'll hear me say: "No is a full sentence. Protect your peace." Say it out loud if you need to. Then circle back to these pages again when life piles on.

My voice in this book is honest, bold, funny, painful, hopeful, and kind. I've been the one crying over spreadsheets and scheduling at midnight, the one in yoga pants sending urgent emails at 2 p.m., the one crawling into bed thinking, "Is this it?" I'm not a zen guru or a Doctor—I'm you.

Let's reclaim your energy, your focus, your humanity—with stories from my life, tools you can use under fluorescent lights or after kids fall asleep, and the permission to laugh, even if it's at how many times you say, "Why am I like this?"

This message is for everyone who's ever felt pressured to hustle harder, prove more, or outfit all the boxes of success. It's for the exhausted caregiver, the driven employee, the solo entrepreneur, the frazzled visionary. Maybe your job loves you—but the pace doesn't. Maybe your passions drive you—but drain you too. This book is your ally when the world says, "Go harder," and you whisper back "Not today."

When you close this intro, here's my hope:

That you feel permission to pause, even if it's five minutes.

That you sense relief in setting a boundary you've been terrified of saying.

That you see this book not as just another self-help title but as a lifeline you'll return to, chapter by chapter, breath by breath, break by break.

My dream is for you to feel human again. Energized again. Whole again.

Flip the page when you're ready. Thousands are already on this journey—and they're still coming back.

With fierce love and unwavering belief in your energy,

Calissa Ngozi

TABLE OF CONTENTS

Dedication & Heart Acknowledgments   IV

MY GIFT TO YOU   VII

My Dream   VIII

Your Health Comes First   XIV

Preface   XV

Reclaiming Our Energy in a World That
Glorifies Exhaustion   XVII

Section One
Oxygen Mask Burnout Recovery Tools (C.A.R.E.)   **1**

    Introduction   2

    Chapter One CLARITY-Mental   5

    Chapter Two ACTIVITY – Physical   12

    Chapter Three RESILIENCE – Emotional   21

    Chapter Four ENGAGEMENT – Social + Spiritual   30

Section Two
What is Self-Care—Really?   **38**

    Chapter Five Self-Care Has Been Watered Down   41

Chapter Six Self-Care ≠ Self-Indulgence   48

Chapter Seven Self-Care Is Maintenance,
Not Rescue   55

Chapter Eight The Four Domains of Self-Care   63

Chapter Nine Self-Care in Real Life
(Not Just on Sundays)   71

Chapter Ten Self-Care Is a Boundary, a Practice,
and a Birthright   78

Section Three
Not Enough Time in the Day?   **86**

Chapter Eleven The Illusion of Time Scarcity   88

Chapter Twelve The Time Trap —
Busy vs. Productive   96

Chapter Thirteen Free (But Powerful) Ways to
Create More Time   104

Chapter Fourteen Restorative Activities That
Don't Cost a Dime   111

Chapter Fifteen The Art of Doing Nothing
(And Why It's Essential)   118

Chapter Sixteen Leveraging the Time You Have
(Even When It Feels Like None)   125

Chapter Seventeen Time Is a Resource—
Use It Wisely   133

Section Four
Putting On Your Mask Daily   **139**

    Chapter Eighteen Marking your Milestones   142

    Chapter Nineteen The Oxygen Mask is a Mindset,
    Not a Moment   148

    Chapter Twenty What Burnout Taught Us
    (And the Permission to Choose Differently)   155

    Chapter Twenty-One But What Happens
    When You're Neuro-Spicy?   163

    Chapter Twenty-Two The Oxygen Mask Mindset—
    An Invitation to Keep Going   170

Author's Note   175

About the Author   178

MY GIFT TO YOU   181

Your Health Comes First

This book is honest. It is bold. It might stir up feelings you have kept tucked away. It might bring up memories or truths you have been carrying quietly for a long time. That is not weakness. That is your body and heart saying, "I am paying attention now."

If at any point these pages feel heavy, I want you to remember the Oxygen Mask Mindset. You do not push through on empty just to get to the end. You pause. You breathe. You care for yourself first so you have what you need to keep going. That might mean putting the book down, getting fresh air, or calling someone who can hold space for you. There is no prize for reading this all at once.

Move at your own pace. Skip around if you need to. Come back to certain pages when you are ready. That is part of the work.

Your health comes first, always. This is not just a gentle reminder. This is your permission slip to treat yourself like the most important person in the room. Because you are.

Preface

"You can't go back and change the beginning, but you can start where you are and change the ending." – C.S. Lewis

---

I was tired, so very tired. We live in a world that glorifies exhaustion. I trained myself and others around me to believe that I was resilient and that I would persevere among any obstacle that came my way. I love keeping busy. I mean, I identify as Neuro-Spicy. Not only do I have ADHD as my superpower, but sometimes my brain likes to sprinkle a little anxiety for good measure.

The name of the game for me was intention and momentum. I was going to become successful—no matter the cost. I was going to create a legacy for the kids I may have one day. I was determined that despite my circumstances growing up, I would go from victim to valour. I would be the voice for the voiceless, the face of what tragedy to triumph looks like. This worked for a little while until it didn't.

It wasn't until I was older that I realized something needed to change in me, or I was going to continue to turn into a person I didn't know.

I want to be used as an example for others who potentially are going through the same circumstances that I did. This book is my love letter to all of those who are tired but willing to put in the work to change their emotional circumstance.

I want you to walk with me hand-in-hand with purpose and intention, with a desire to unpack what society has told us. I want you to put yourselves first. Walk with me on this journey so we can define what unlearning burnout, redefining resilience, and choosing yourself really means. Allow me to teach you that there is recovery after trying to hold it all together.

Reclaiming Our Energy in a World That Glorifies Exhaustion

aka The Hard Truth You Already Knew but Needed to Hear Louder...

Let's just get one thing straight from the jump: This world will gladly take every drop of your energy—and still ask for more.

That's not drama. That's the design.

We are living in a system that rewards overworking, celebrates burnout as ambition, and hands out gold stars for self-abandonment. "She never stops!" they say, like it's a compliment. We get applause for sacrificing our time, health, and peace. But the moment we slow down? Set a boundary? Say, "No, I'm actually going to rest now," we're immediately questioned, judged, or made to feel guilty.

And we've internalized it. We wear our exhaustion like a badge of honor.

We say things like:

"I'm just so busy" as if that proves we're valuable.

"I'll rest when things calm down" (spoiler: they won't).

Or my personal favorite, "I'm fine,"
when we're clearly falling apart inside.

Let's call it what it is: burnout in a cute outfit.

We've been trained to confuse being needed with being worthy.

We've been taught that our energy exists for other people to consume.

And we've been fed the lie that the only way to succeed is to run ourselves into the ground.

But here's the thing: that narrative is not only broken—it's dangerous, and it's time we stop agreeing to it.

This Book Is a Wake-Up Call (Not a Whisper)

You didn't pick up this book because life was working just fine.

You picked it up because something inside you-maybe tired, maybe fed up, maybe whispering through clenched teeth, said: There has to be another way.

Well guess what. There is.

But let's be clear: choosing yourself in a world that benefits from you burning out is not an easy choice. It's not always going to feel good or clean or Instagrammable. It might look like saying "no" to things people expect you to say "yes" to. It might mean disappointing folks who were just fine with you constantly putting yourself last.

But that discomfort? That friction? That's you reclaiming your power.

That's you interrupting the script you were handed—and writing a new one that starts with this:

> My energy is mine. My time is mine. My peace is mine. And I'm not sorry for protecting them.

The World Will Not Hand You Rest-You Have to Take It

Let me be real: nobody is going to come save you from burnout.

Not your boss.
Not your family.
Not the system.
Not even your group chat.

They're too used to you being the one who "always handles it."

They're too comfortable with the version of you who never says no.

They're not evil—they're just used to your overgiving.

But they don't get to decide what you need anymore. You do.

So let me ask you this:

What would your life look like if you stopped asking for permission to rest?

What if you started treating your energy like the sacred, powerful, non-renewable resource it is?

What if you finally believed that you don't have to prove your worth by running on empty?

This book is going to walk you through how. Not with fluff. Not with vague self-care platitudes. But with a bold, honest framework that will help you shift your mindset, reclaim your time, and get radically clear on your needs.

We'll laugh a bit. Reflect a lot. I'll share the times I didn't choose myself, and the powerful moments I finally did. I'll hand you tools you can actually use, not just feel inspired by. Because this isn't about becoming a better version of yourself; it's about becoming the most true version of yourself.

The one who doesn't hustle for worth.

The one who sets boundaries like it's a love language.

The one who rests without guilt, says no without apology, and breathes without asking.

Here's Your First Truth Bomb:

You're not exhausted because you're weak.

You're exhausted because you've been strong for too damn long.

And now?

You get to do something different.

You get to stop glorifying exhaustion and start honoring your energy.

You get to put your oxygen mask on first, and not feel one ounce of shame about it.

A Few Questions Before We Begin:

- When did I first learn that being exhausted meant I was doing enough?

- What parts of my identity are tied to being constantly busy or available?

- What would it mean for me to reclaim my energy— without apology?

Write these down. Sit with them. Let them linger. You don't have to have the answers yet. But the fact that you're here means you're ready to start asking.

Final Thought – Oxygen Mask Moment

The oxygen mask framework isn't a moment. It's a mindset.

And it starts right now.

Welcome to The Oxygen Mask Mindset. Let's begin.

Section One
Oxygen Mask Burnout Recovery Tools (C.A.R.E.)

"I can be changed by what happens to me, but I refuse to be reduced by it." – Maya Angelou

Introduction

You Cannot Pour from an Empty Bucket. The time it took me not only to truly understand this notion but to embrace it at full value admittedly took longer than it should have. I am a work in progress.

I was in my early 20s and I can honestly remember it like it was yesterday. I was newly married, working 4 jobs and going to school full-time. I would work 11pm-7am at a residential group home for behavioral teens, then I would go home and shower and rush off to school. After my classes, I would sleep from 12pm-230pm before rushing to the after-school program. I would then go to the McDonalds drive through and then race to the evening program at one of 2 rec centres. I would go home and shower, then head back to my night shift (awake job) and repeat the cycle for an entire year. I would average 2-3 hours of sleep a night, 5 days a week. On weekends I got a little reprieve, and it was closer to 5-6 hours of sleep. I felt like I had nothing to lose and everything to gain. I was madly in love. I was young, determined, and confident. I had everything to gain and nothing to lose—until I almost did.

One night after a year of my gruelling schedule, I was lying on my husband's lap in the living room, and I completely broke down. I lied there, sobbing uncontrollably. My husband was patient with me until I was ready to talk. I looked up at him and simply said I can't continue to live like this. I'm going to end up in the hospital with a mental health crisis. It's important to note here that I am not someone who likes to share their emotions with anyone. It is one of my protective layers: trying to escape vulnerability.

I wasn't working all of these jobs simply for financial gain. My determination and grit did not turn into resilience. I put myself in this position for many reasons, one of them being my thought process (and admittedly my stubbornness). *If I just keep at it, my resume is going to look spectacular and I'll be able to land any job my heart desires.* You see, at this time and place in my life, I had a really hard time saying no to job opportunities. It didn't translate into feelings of being overwhelmed; I felt it was connected to my greater purpose, which at that time I couldn't even identify. My husband looked at me and told me, "You don't have to continue to do this. Your mental health is worth so much more." After that conversation, I quit two of my jobs and never looked back.

Burnout cannot be categorized as just exhaustion. It is the feeling of depletion across many parts of us. Today, we live in a world that glorifies exhaustion. We are led to believe that the only way to succeed in life is to participate in the constant grind. To chase after our goals no matter the cost to ourselves personally and professionally. The notion of taking a break, vacation, or time to pause and reflect is often looked down upon. Not only in professional settings, but at home as well.

The moment I realized that you cannot be everything to everyone all the time is the birthplace of my concept, The Oxygen Mask Mindset™. It is the realization that self-care and setting boundaries is not a luxury. It is necessary in order for us to live fully with minimal stress. Over the next few chapters, we will break down my C.A.R.E. Tool (Clarity, Activity, Resilience, Engagement) and really dive into how it can help re-wire our thinking when it comes to understanding burnout and the importance of self-care. We will unpack the lies that we've not only been told but that we tell ourselves and each other in trying to justify overworking and overwhelming ourselves.

Chapter One
CLARITY-Mental

"You can't read the label from inside the jar."
– Unknown

That quote shook me the first time I heard it. Because it was *me*. I was moving so fast, doing all the things, achieving all the goals—but I couldn't see what I was becoming. I couldn't hear myself think. I couldn't remember what I even *wanted* anymore.

This chapter is about the mental clutter that builds when you've been going for too long without a pause. When your brain is stuck in overdrive and your thoughts are so tangled, you can't separate what's real from what's just noise.

Clarity is the first part of the C.A.R.E. Tool because it's the foundation. If you can't get clear, you can't make empowered decisions. You can't say no to the things draining you, and you definitely can't say yes to what gives you life.

When Your Brain Feels Like a Browser with 42 Tabs Open

Have you ever stood in the middle of a room and forgotten why you walked in there? Or tried to write an email and ended up staring at a blinking cursor for 30 minutes? That's not just "being tired." That's mental burnout.

In my worst burnout moments, I wasn't just tired. I was foggy. Irritable. Disconnected. I was so overwhelmed that I couldn't focus on a single thought long enough to make a decision. I would overanalyze the smallest things—like what to make for dinner, or how to word a text—and then beat myself up for not being more efficient.

And here's the thing: no one else could see it. I was still showing up. Still working. Still smiling.

But inside? I was screaming for silence.

I remember one night in particular. I had spent the entire day trying to catch up on everything—emails, groceries, housework, calls—and still felt like I had accomplished *nothing*. I sat on the couch, turned on a show I had been looking forward to and realized I couldn't even follow the plot. My brain was too full. Not with deep thoughts or feelings, but just static. Noise.

What Mental Burnout Really Looks Like

Let's name it, because clarity starts with language.

When you're mentally burnt out, it might look like:

- **Brain fog**: That fuzzy, disconnected feeling when everything feels *harder* than it should be.

- **Forgetfulness**: Missing appointments, repeating stories, forgetting words mid-sentence.

- **Decision fatigue**: Feeling paralyzed by simple choices—like what to wear or what to eat.

- **Racing thoughts but low output**: Constantly thinking, but getting very little done.

- **Inner spirals**: Ruminating over the past, obsessing about the future, doubting yourself at every turn.

We live in a world that encourages constant stimulation—scrolling, comparing, working, doing. But the human brain wasn't designed for nonstop input. Clarity begins when we honor our limits instead of pushing past them.

My Personal Turning Point

There was a time I thought being busy equaled being important. I used to say yes to every opportunity because I didn't want to miss out (I still struggle with this). Because I thought saying no meant I was lazy or ungrateful. Because I tied my worth to my output.

But eventually, my brain said, "Enough."

I was in a meeting, listening to someone talk, and I suddenly realized I hadn't absorbed a single word they'd said in the last 10 minutes. I was nodding, but my mind was somewhere else entirely. Not because I didn't care—but because I had nothing left to give. My brain was full of worry, to-do lists, and emotional exhaustion. That was a wake-up call.

Tools That Help Clear the Clutter

Let's talk about what you can actually *do* when you're mentally overloaded. These aren't magic solutions—but they're gentle shifts that help bring you back to yourself.

1. Mind-Dumping/Journaling

This is my number one go-to. Mind-dumping is just writing down or voice noting *everything* that's swirling in your brain. No structure, no grammar rules, no filter. It's like taking a broom to your thoughts and sweeping them out of your head and onto the page.

I usually set a timer for 10 minutes and just let it all out: worries, tasks, fears, frustrations, random reminders. When I do this regularly, I feel *lighter*. Like I can finally breathe.

Don't worry about sounding wise or profound. Just be honest.

Try this: Start with the phrase "Right now, I'm thinking about..." and go from there.

2. "No-Thought" Spaces

Sometimes your brain doesn't need more thinking. It needs *less*.

Enter what I call "no-thought" spaces—quiet moments when you give yourself full permission *not* to be productive. This could be a walk in nature, lying on the floor and listening to music, watching the clouds, or sitting on your balcony with your phone on airplane mode.

I try to build these moments into my day, even if it's just five minutes. They're not wasted time—they're *recovery time*. Think of it as a rest stop on a long drive. Without it, you'll miss your destination entirely.

3. Micro-Decisions

Mental burnout often comes from decision overload. So when you're in the thick of it, reduce the number of choices you have to make.

Wear the same outfit on repeat (although this one might actually stress me out).

Prep the same lunch all week.

Default to "no" unless something feels like a *true* yes.

Micro-decisions conserve mental energy. The goal isn't to control everything—it's to simplify enough that you can *think clearly again*.

4. Recognizing Neurodivergence

I'll be real with you: as someone who has ADHD, a lot of traditional self-care advice has never worked for me. Telling me to "just focus" or "prioritize better" is like telling a fish to climb a tree.

What helped me was learning to work *with* my brain, not against it. I started scheduling things in short sprints. I gave myself permission to rest without guilt. I used color coding and timers and sticky notes and a whole lot of compassion.

If your brain works differently, your recovery will too—and that's not a flaw. That's your superpower in disguise.

Reflection Prompt

Where do my thoughts spiral when I'm burnt out?

Do you spiral into shame? Fear letting people down? Obsess over what you "should" be doing?

Write it down. Speak it out loud. Share it with someone you trust.

Naming the spiral is how you break it.

Final Thoughts – Oxygen Mask Moment: Clarity Isn't Perfection—It's Permission

Let me be clear: clarity doesn't mean you'll have everything figured out. It doesn't mean you'll never forget something again or that your mind will be peaceful 24/7.

Clarity is about permission.

Permission to stop.

Permission to breathe.

Permission to be honest about what your brain and heart actually need.

You don't have to hustle for your worth. You don't have to do it all to be enough. You just have to show up for yourself—one small, clear step at a time.

So if you're feeling foggy right now, I want you to know: that fog will lift. It always does. Especially when you make space for clarity to return.

Let's move forward, gently.

Chapter Two
ACTIVITY – Physical

Real Talk Tip: "Your body remembers everything your brain tries to forget." – JL Moreno

---

Before I knew what burnout was, I thought I was just "someone who got sick a lot."

Every few weeks, like clockwork, I'd come down with something—a cold, a sinus infection, an upset stomach, sometimes even a migraine that would knock me out for a day or two and require prescribed medication. I'd take a sick day, load up on lemon tea and cough drops, oregano oil, orange juice, vitamin C—ALL the things. I would pop some Advil, try to sleep it off, and then get right back to the grind.

I told myself I just had a "sensitive immune system." Or that it was the weather. Or that I was around too many people. What I didn't realize was that I wasn't just catching colds—I was breaking down. My body wasn't betraying me. It was trying to save me.

At the time, I was in go-mode 24/7. Multiple jobs. School deadlines. A new marriage. Emotional caretaking. My brain was always on, and I treated my body like an after-thought—something that would just keep up because I needed it to.

But eventually, my body had had enough.

It was trying to tell me the only way it knew how:

"I'm tired. I need care. I need attention."

But I wasn't listening until the symptoms forced me to slow down.

Looking back, I realize I didn't need more Vitamin C. I needed rest.

I didn't need another over-the-counter fix. I needed to reconnect with myself.

And that's what this chapter is really about.

What Physical Burnout Really Looks Like

Let's name it. Let's name it without shame.

When you're physically burned out, it might look like:

- Waking up tired, no matter how many hours you slept

- Tension headaches that start before breakfast

- Digestive issues with no clear diagnosis (bloating, cramping, IBS-like symptoms)

- Muscle aches and body pain for "no reason"

- Restlessness at night, but exhaustion during the day

- Constant jaw clenching, shallow breathing, and a nervous system that lives on high alert

You might think you just need more coffee. A better pillow. A different workout plan.

But what your body might be asking for is **relief**. Regulation. A chance to exhale fully.

You can't think your way out of burnout—you have to move through it. Literally. That means movement that heals. Stillness that restores. Food that fuels. Rest that resets.

My Body Was the Last to Give Up-and the First to Break

I used to say, "My body just pushes through." I wore it like a badge of honor. I had conditioned myself to believe that aches, fatigue, and tension were just the price of ambition.

I didn't realize I was running on adrenaline.

And here's the kicker: for a while, it worked. I was highly functional. Productive. Smiling. Saying yes to everything. I thought I was thriving.

Until one day I wasn't.

I remember walking into a room and forgetting why I was there. I remember sitting in a meeting and feeling like I was floating above my own body, detached and dizzy. I was so used to being exhausted, I didn't even recognize the warning signs anymore. But my body did.

It wasn't until my stomach started rejecting food, my chest tightened daily, and I started having mini panic episodes at night that I realized something had to give.

Activity stopped being a checkbox. It became a lifeline.

Rebuilding Connection Through Activity

This isn't about doing more. It's about reconnecting. Healing your relationship with your body through intentional, caring movement and rest.

Let's break it down.

1. Regulate Before You "Motivate"

You don't need more hustle. You need regulation.

When your nervous system is in survival mode, no amount of journaling or yoga or productivity hacks will fix it. You're not lazy. You're dysregulated.

Burnout puts your body in a constant state of fight, flight, freeze—or fawn. That's a trauma response, not a personal flaw.

Regulation techniques that help me:

- **Breathwork**: Start with box breathing (inhale for 4, hold for 4, exhale for 4, hold for 4). It calms the body like nothing else.

- **Progressive muscle relaxation**: Tense and re- lease each muscle group slowly, from your feet to your face.

- **Cold water therapy**: Splashing cold water on your face can instantly ground you by activating the va- gus nerve.

- **Somatic shaking**: Sounds strange, but shaking your limbs (like animals do after stress) can dis- charge nervous energy.

None of these things take long—but they start rewiring your sense of safety in your body. When you're safe, you can heal.

2. Redefine "Movement"

Let's throw away the guilt-laced definition of exercise. You don't owe anyone a certain number of steps or reps or calories burned (who came up with 10,000 steps a day anyways?). You owe your body joy.

Movement doesn't have to mean a workout. It can be:

- Walking while listening to music that reminds you of who you are

- Stretching slowly in bed in the morning with deep breaths

- Dancing around your living room with no one watching

- Rolling your neck, opening your chest, swinging your arms

- Taking the stairs slowly and noticing your body moving with intention

Sometimes I put on a playlist and move my body the way it wants to move—not the way a fitness app tells me to. That is sacred. That is healing.

Joyful movement counts. In fact, it counts more when you're recovering from burnout.

3. Sleep Isn't Lazy—It's Essential

Can we say this louder for the people in the back?

SLEEP IS NOT A LUXURY.

It is the foundation of mental, emotional, and physical health. If you're not sleeping well, everything else will feel harder than it needs to.

And yet, in burnout culture, sleep is often the first thing sacrificed. Late-night emails. Doomscrolling. Working "after hours." Sleep is treated like something you have to earn, instead of something you deserve just for being human.

If you're waking up exhausted, here's what might help:

- **Wind-down rituals**: Give your brain cues that it's time to rest—dim lights, calming music, or gentle stretches.

- **A no-tech bedtime buffer**: Try 30 minutes tech-free before sleep. Let your brain unplug.

- **Cognitive offloading**: Write your to-dos or racing thoughts down before bed so they don't stay swirling in your head.

- **Nervous system support**: Herbal tea, magnesium, calming scents like lavender—these signal safety to your body.

You don't need to "deserve" sleep. You require it. Prioritize it without apology.

4. Fuel Without Shame

This is a tender one. Because burnout often comes with body shame. And when you're trying to reconnect with yourself, food can be loaded with guilt, pressure, or even control.

But your body cannot recover from burnout if it is starving, physically or emotionally.

Here's what I've learned:

- Eat regularly. Even when you're not "hungry" in the typical way and especially when you're emotionally depleted.

- Hydrate. Add some electrolytes or fruit to your water if you need to make it feel like care.

- Give yourself permission to eat what you enjoy. Stop punishing your body for being tired. Nourish it like you would someone you love.

There is no one-size-fits-all food plan.

There is only listening.

Your Body Has Been Speaking to You All Along

You've been taught to push through. To keep going. To ignore the pain.

But what if the tension in your neck wasn't just about bad posture?

What if the gut issues weren't just food sensitivity, but *life sensitivity*?

What if your body wasn't breaking down, but *begging to be heard*?

The body always tells the truth. The beautiful part is: it also remembers safety, softness, and strength. It knows how to come back from the edge—if we let it.

Reflection Prompts

- Where is my body holding tension right now?

- What does movement look like when it feels joyful, not forced?

- What would it look like to let rest be a right— not a reward?

Final Thoughts – Oxygen Mask Moment: Your Body Is Not the Problem. It's the Messenger.

Your body isn't working against you. It's working for you, every single second.

Even when it's tired. Even when it's aching. Even when it's screaming for rest.

Activity isn't about pushing harder. It's about learning to move, rest, nourish, and listen to your body in a way that builds trust.

This is a new rhythm. A gentler pace. A more compassion-ate relationship with the skin you're in.

The world will keep spinning. You don't have to.

Let yourself be still. Let yourself move. Let yourself feel.

Let your body be a *place of healing*, not just survival.

Let's keep going-not harder, but deeper. Next, we'll talk about the emotional weight we carry, and how to start building true resilience, not just survival.

Chapter Three
RESILIENCE - Emotional

Mantra: "All of me is welcome here—even the messy parts."
– Unknown

For the longest time, I thought "resilience" meant pushing through.

I thought it meant staying calm in the chaos, never showing emotion, showing up with it all together, even when I was crumbling inside. I thought it meant being "the strong one"—the one who held it all together for everyone else. Who could listen to everyone's problems and still smile. Who could keep performing under pressure like it didn't cost her anything.

But it was costing me. It just wasn't showing up as one big breakdown. It was slow. It was quiet.

And it started with feeling numb.

The Emotionally Burned-Out Version of Me

I remember sitting across from a friend at brunch. They were telling me a hilarious story about something that had happened at work-and I was laughing on the outside. I was fully engaged. Like, full smile, making all the right sounds. I was selling it! But inside?

Nothing.

I felt flat. Disconnected. Like I was watching a version of myself perform being "fine." I was really good at it too, until I wasn't.

I didn't feel joy. I didn't feel much of anything. And that scared me more than sadness ever had. What was happening to me?

There was a time when I was all feelings. I'd cry at movies, light up over new ideas, get butterflies before big opportunities. But burnout muted everything. My emotions got blurry, like a photo out of focus. And when they did come through, they were loud and unpredictable: tears out of nowhere, becoming easily triggered with the people I loved, anxiety that clung to me like static. I was unraveling at a rapid pace.

I was falling apart. I didn't know if I was ever going to climb off this emotional rollercoaster I was riding.

What I've come to understand is this: I wasn't falling apart—I was emotionally overloaded, overstimulated, and undersupported.

I wasn't weak. I was tired. I was stretched past my capacity. I felt like I had absolutely nothing left in me.

How Emotional Burnout Shows Up

Let's name it, without shame. Emotional burnout might look like:

- Being so irritated (triggered) over something small, but not understanding why

- Crying in the car, or not being able to cry at all

- Avoiding social events, preferred activities, calls or texts because you don't have the energy to "be on"

- Feeling like your moods are unpredictable and hard to explain

- Snapping at your kids, your partner, your coworkers—and then spiraling in guilt

- Zoning out during things you used to love because joy feels far away

- Feeling like you're living life behind a glass wall, watching but not really living

Maybe you've thought, I don't even recognize myself.

Maybe you've wondered, Where did my joy go?

I want you to know this: your emotions are not broken. They are overwhelmed. They need space, not shame.

Emotional Resilience is a Practice, Not a Trait

We think some people are just born with more emotional resilience. That they're naturally stronger, more stable, more positive. But that's not the full truth.

Resilience is not a personality type—it's a skill. One you can learn how to nurture. One that gets stronger when it's fed with compassion, self-awareness, and safe spaces.

It starts with allowing yourself to *feel*, even when it's uncomfortable.

Let's break this down into practical tools that can help you rebuild emotional strength without bypassing your very real experience.

Practices to Support Emotional Resilience

1. Do Regular Emotional Check-Ins

I'll be honest—this felt awkward at first. Asking myself "What am I feeling?" when I could barely make it through my day felt like a luxury I didn't have time for.

But the truth is, I couldn't afford not to ask!

Burnout disconnects you from your emotional self. Staying disconnected only prolongs the suffering that you are going through.

So now, I ask myself a few times a day:

- *What am I feeling?*

- *Where do I feel it in my body?*

- *What do I need right now, if anything?*

Sometimes the answer is, *I don't know.* That's okay. Naming the confusion is still a sense of connection.

This is how you are going to start the slow rebuild. The tender return to who you are.

2. Name It to Move It

Emotions that stay unnamed stay stuck!

Think of your feelings like houseguests. If you don't answer the door, they just bang louder. But when you name them—"Hey, anxiety. Hey, trauma, Hey, anger."—they soften. They don't have to scream to get your attention.

You can:

- Say the emotion out loud

- Journal a few lines about where it's coming from

- Use a voice note to let it out without needing to "make sense"

You don't need a therapist's couch to begin this work (though therapy is always welcome here and encouraged). You just need honesty.

3. Create Safe Emotional Release

If you're holding emotional tension in your body—and let's be real, most of us are—you need outlets that feel safe and unfiltered.

That might mean:

- Screaming into a pillow (this is one of my go-tos)

- Crying in the shower (or while watching emotional Youtube and TikTok videos)

- Blasting music in your car and singing until your throat hurts (and maybe the tears flow)

- Journaling the stuff you never say out loud (and may need to burn after reading)

- Moving your body in a way that matches the energy (stomping, swaying, shaking it out)

Another one of my go-to practices? I record voice memos when I'm upset. No filter. Just the messy muddle of my feelings. I don't always listen back. Sometimes I delete them right after. But just saying it out loud moves something. I exhale.

There is power in expression without performance.

4. Protect Your Emotional Energy with Boundaries

This isn't just about saying "no" to tasks. It's about saying "no" to dynamics that drain you.

If someone leaves you feeling emotionally wrung out every time you interact, that's a clue. If you always feel guilty after hanging up the phone with someone, that's a clue. If your calendar is full but your soul feels empty, that's a big clue.

You're allowed to:

- Delay responding

- Say, "I'm not available for this conversation right now"

- Set limits on your giving, especially when you're running on fumes

- Unfollow, mute, or take breaks from things that overstimulate or upset you

Boundaries don't make you selfish.

They make you sustainable.

Mantra Check-In

All of me is welcome here—even the messy parts.

Even the version of you that didn't get anything done today.

Even the part of you that snapped at your kids or your partner and felt horrible after.

Even the version that's "fine" on the outside but silently spiraling inside.

You don't have to hide your sadness. You don't have to disguise your happiness.

You don't have to tone yourself down to be what you think other people want you to be.

You get to be all of you. Fully. Freely. Unapologetically. You.

That's what healing looks like.

Reflection Prompts

- What emotions do I *dismiss* or *downplay* most often?

- What makes me feel emotionally safe?

- When was the last time I felt emotionally *stable*— and what helped me get there?

Final Thoughts – Oxygen Mask Moment: You Don't Need to Be Tough to Be Resilient

Somewhere along the way, we learned that strength meant silence. That being "strong" meant being unfazed, unbothered, untouchable.

The world taught us to push through pain. To keep smiling. To "stay positive."

But emotional resilience isn't about pretending you're okay. It's about becoming someone who can sit with discomfort and still feel worthy.

But here's what I know now:

The strongest people I've ever met are the ones who feel deeply and keep showing up with intention.

The ones who say, "This is hard, and I'm still choosing to care for myself."

The ones who cry, rest, fall apart—and get back up softer, not harder.

You are not here to be emotionally bulletproof. You are here to be emotionally honest.

And honesty, my friend, is a form of power that you can take back!

Chapter Four
ENGAGEMENT – Social + Spiritual

Oxygen Mask Check-In Prompt: "Which area of the C.A.R.E. Tool—Clarity, Activity, Resilience, or Engagement—needs my oxygen today?"

Burnout doesn't just drain your energy. It drains your ability to feel connected, to people, to purpose, and sometimes even to yourself.

When we're in survival mode, life becomes transactional. Conversations. Relationships. Even happiness can start to feel like one more thing to "schedule." But connection isn't just a luxury—it's essential to healing.

You weren't designed to go through life numb, distant, or isolated.

You were made for **Engagement**. For meaning. For moments of softness and togetherness that refill you from the inside out.

We will continue to relate back, but this final chapter in the **C.A.R.E. Tool** section of this book is about reclaiming that connection—without pressure, without guilt, and without the performance we're so often used to putting on.

Disengagement Doesn't Always Look Like Isolation

Here's something I had to learn the hard way: burnout in your engagement area doesn't always look like being alone. Sometimes you're surrounded by people, places, and things, but still feel completely disconnected from all of it!

You show up to work. You check in on your group chats. You do all the things. But it feels empty. Like you're floating through scenes in a favorite movie you no longer want to watch.

That's burnout in your Engagement. It is a disconnection from what lights you up and grounds you.

Often it shows up subtly—through irritability, apathy, or an aching sense of "What's even the point?"

Signs of Burnout in Your Engagement

- You feel distant from your friends, family, or community

- Conversations feel like effort and not nourishment

- You dread social interaction but, at the same time, also feel lonely

- You've lost interest in things that used to bring you joy or purpose

- You're craving connection but don't want to reach out

- You feel disconnected from your beliefs, purpose, or creative spark

If any of that feels familiar, you're not broken—you're burned out. And your engagement system is sending out an SOS.

Tools to Reclaim Your Engagement

Engagement doesn't have to mean "being more social." It means creating intentional, nurturing, soul-filling connections—to people, to yourself, to something bigger than your schedule.

Let's talk about what that can look like in practice.

1. Engage With Yourself First

Your Clarity tool is all about getting mentally grounded— but Engagement is how you emotionally and spiritually return to yourself.

That could look like:

- Taking 10 minutes to be fully present—no phone, no noise

- Asking yourself, "What part of me have I been ignoring?"

- Sitting with your favorite music, doing nothing but being present

- Reconnecting with routines: journaling, prayer, tea in silence, reading

Before you can feel reconnected to the world, you have to feel reconnected to you. And that takes intention—not perfection.

2. Build Connection That Nourishes, Not Depletes

You don't need a packed calendar to feel socially engaged! What you need is quality. Realness. Safe spaces.

Engagement might look like:

- Sending a "thinking of you" message to one friend who really gets you

- Having a low-energy hangout where you don't have to talk much

- Laughing over nothing in particular with your chosen family

- Letting someone hold space for your truth, even if it's messy

Remember: you don't have to be "on" to be loved. The right people want the real you—not the filtered version. Those are your people.

3. Engage Spiritually—In Whatever Way Feels Right to You

This is where your Resilience (emotional health) and Engagement intersect. Because when you're feeling emotionally depleted, spiritual grounding can help you make sense of the noise.

For me, my connection to God is what helps me, but I understand that everyone has a different belief system and some none at all. That's okay.

You don't need to be religious to be spiritual. You don't need a perfect meditation practice. You just need something that reconnects you to the bigger picture.

That might be:

- Sitting under a tree and letting yourself breathe

- Lighting a candle and setting an intention

- Talking to your higher power if you have one (for me this is God)

- Reading and listening to things that remind you you're not alone

- Journaling what your soul needs—not what your calendar says

Engagement isn't always loud or active. Sometimes, it's being in solitude and remembering who you are and what still matters.

4. Set Boundaries That Protect Your Engagement

If you're saying yes to everything but feel more disconnected than ever, it's time to check in with your boundaries.

Healthy Engagement doesn't mean constant access. It means aligned access.

You're allowed to:

- Take breaks from group chats

- Cancel without guilt when you need solitude

- Mute the noise (digitally and emotionally) so you can hear your own voice

- Be able to intentionally decide where your energy goes

Boundaries aren't about disconnection. They're how you create the conditions for real connection on your own terms, for your own well-being.

You're Not Just Tired—You're Depleted.

And that means you don't just need rest.

You need *C.A.R.E.*—Clarity, Activity, Resilience, and Engagement.

These tools aren't checkboxes. They're *lifelines*. They're how you reclaim your breath, your boundaries, your being. Healing is not linear. But it is possible.

With each pause. With each choice to care. With each oxygen mask moment.

Check-In Prompt

"Which part of my C.A.R.E. tool—Clarity, Activity, Resilience, or Engagement—needs my oxygen today?"

Ask it often.

Trust the answer.

Respond with care.

You're not starting over.

You're starting again—this time, with yourself at the center.

Reflection Prompts

- Where in my life do I feel most engaged right now? Least engaged?

- Who or what makes me feel emotionally and spiritually grounded?

- What kind of connection am I craving—social, creative, spiritual?

Final Thoughts – Oxygen Mask Moment

"All of me is welcome here—even the messy parts."

Even the version of you who ghosted your group chat.

Even the part of you that wants deep conversation but has no energy to start one.

Even the you that misses your old spark, and wonders whether it's gone forever.

It's not gone. It's just been buried under an immense amount of burnout. And now, we're gently digging your happiness back up.

Section Two
What is Self-Care—Really?

What Self-Care Really Looks Like When You're Burnt Out, Busy, or Barely Holding On

Let's be honest: the word self-care has been THROUGH it.

It's been tossed around in every direction. We have turned it into a hashtag, packaged it into products. We have glorified, oversimplified, and, in many ways, misunderstood its true meaning and intention.

By the time most of us reach the point of burnout, self-care can feel like just another thing we're failing at. Another task. Another performance. Another expectation we can't meet.

But here's what I want to say loud and clear as we begin this section:

- Self-care is not a luxury. It is not a treat. It is not optional.

- Self-care is survival, and for some of us, it's reclamation. It's resistance. It's a return to self in a world that keeps asking us to abandon ourselves.

This section is for the people who are exhausted but still showing up.

For the parents, the leaders, the helpers, the givers—the ones who are tired of hearing "just take care of yourself" without any guidance on what that actually means when you're overwhelmed, under-resourced, or at your limit.

In the next few chapters, we're going to unpack the real face of self-care. Not the curated version. Not the Pinterest mood board. But the gritty, daily, often messy practice of choosing yourself in small, meaningful, powerful ways.

We're going to break through the myths and marketing and talk about what self-care really looks like when you're burnt out, busy, or barely holding on.

So let's start at the beginning.

Chapter Five
Self-Care Has Been
Watered Down

"Caring for myself is not self-indulgence,
it is self-preservation." – Audre Lorde

There's a reason I hesitated before using the phrase self-care in this book.

Because let's be honest, it's been branded to death.

Self-care has been turned into a mood board. A product. A checklist. A perfectly filtered reel of someone else's ideal morning routine that, if we're being real, only works if you're already well-rested, well-funded, and not in the middle of a mental breakdown.

And while I love a good lavender and eucalyptus candle, a mani/pedi, a facial and a 90-minute massage, that is not what saved me when I was at my lowest.

When I was deep in burnout? When I was working four jobs, sleeping two hours a night, feeling disconnected from my body and my joy? No number of bubble baths or jade rollers were going to help.

Because self-care has been watered down. And in doing so, we've lost sight of what it's actually supposed to do.

Self-Care Has Become Something We Buy, Not Something We Do

There's a difference between comfort and care. Comfort feels good in the moment. Care goes deeper.

You can buy comfort. You can click "add to cart" and feel that little dopamine rush from ordering something that promises ease. You can light that $90 candle and sip tea from the mug with the affirmations on it—and still feel like you're unraveling inside.

I've done it. I've performed self-care like a role I was auditioning for.

I've sat in clean sweatpants, wearing a face mask, journaling with expensive pens... and still felt like I was crumbling.

Because none of those things fix burnout. They might soothe it temporarily. But if self-care stops at the surface, we're just decorating the chaos. Not healing it.

Self-Care Can't Be a Reward for Suffering

This one hits hard:

Self-care has been twisted into something we earn.

We tell ourselves:

- "I can rest after I finish this project."

- "I'll take time off when things slow down."

- "Once I prove I'm doing enough, then I'll take care of myself."

But here's the truth no one tells you:

Things won't slow down on their own.

The world doesn't hand out breaks. It rewards burnout. It celebrates the grind. We live in a world that glorifies exhaustion.

If you're waiting for permission to care for yourself, you'll wait forever.

Self-care isn't a treat.

It's not a bonus.

It's a survival strategy.

What Self-Care Really Looks Like in the Mess

Let's normalize what self-care can actually look like when you're burnt out, busy, or just over everything and everyone:

- Saying "I can't" even though people expect you to show up

- Lying on the floor in silence for 15 minutes because that's all you can do

- Ignoring laundry and dishes because your brain is already overstimulated

- Choosing sleep instead of staying up to catch up on life

- Ordering takeout without judgment

- Not explaining why you're unavailable— and refusing to apologize for it

Real self-care isn't always cute. It's often inconvenient. It disrupts the expectations that others have placed on us— and the ones we've placed on ourselves.

Self-Care Is Not Selfish

Let me be clear: there's a reason people feel guilty about self-care.

Because we were raised—especially those of us from marginalized or high-responsibility communities—to believe that worth is earned through output. That sacrifice is noble. That exhaustion is honorable. That rest is lazy. That needing help is weakness.

So when we slow down, even a little, the guilt creeps in.

It whispers, other people don't get to rest. Who do you think you are?

It tells us that boundaries are mean, that rest is indulgent, and that "doing nothing" is failure.

But here's the thing: *you don't owe anyone your burnout!*

You don't have to torch yourself to keep others warm.

You don't have to be everything to everyone to be valuable.

You don't have to suffer in silence just to make others comfortable.

Self-care isn't selfish. It's how we stay alive in a world that keeps asking for more.

Sometimes Self-Care Is Choosing You—Even When Others Don't Like It

I want to say this as clearly as I can: Self-care is not always soft. Sometimes it's savage.

It's cancelling. Walking away. Saying no. Closing the laptop. Not answering the text. Not explaining your no. Disappointing someone and letting them sit with it.

Sometimes self-care is messy, fierce, disruptive.

Sometimes it looks like:

- Quitting something you once fought for

- Saying, "I'm not available for that conversation anymore"

- Unfollowing accounts that make you feel inadequate

- Leaving events early

- Letting go of people who only love you when you're useful

That's not cruelty. That's clarity. That's boundaries in motion.

That's care.

Redefining Self-Care as a Practice, Not a Performance

You don't need a checklist. You need choice.

Real self-care is not one-size-fits-all. It's dynamic. It changes based on your needs, your season, your capacity.

So instead of asking:

"What should I be doing for self-care?"

Ask yourself:

- What part of me is craving care right now?

- Am I trying to perform care or actually experience it?

- What would it look like to care for myself like I matter?

This isn't about being perfect. It's about being present—to your needs, your limits, and your humanity.

Reflection Prompts

- When have I treated self-care like a luxury instead of a necessity?

- What kinds of "performative" self-care do I do out of guilt, not love?

- What would it look like to practice self-care without shame or permission?

Real Talk Reminder

You don't have to wait for burnout to give yourself care.

You don't have to collapse to finally cancel.

You don't have to cry to realize you've done too much.

You are allowed to choose yourself before the breaking point.

Because you deserve care now—not when you've earned it.

Not when you've hit a wall. Not when you've finally "proven" how tired you are.

Chapter Six
Self-Care ≠ Self-Indulgence

Truth Bomb: "Resting doesn't make you weak.
It makes you ready."

Let's go ahead and break this WIDE open:

Taking care of yourself is not selfish. It is not extra. And it is definitely not indulgent.

I say this with love AND fire—because the world has worked hard to convince us otherwise.

Especially if you were raised to believe that being strong meant being needed.

Especially if you've carried a family, a job, a community, or your own survival on your back.

Especially if you've been taught that your value lives in what you can do for other people.

There's a special kind of guilt that shows up when you try to choose yourself after years of being the reliable one. The strong one. The one who keeps it all together.

This was and is a continued struggle for me that I have had to learn how to overcome. I always felt like I had to be at 100% for everything and everyone—except for myself. This is one of the reasons I wrote this book. To dismantle not only societal expectations of me but the ones I had for myself. I had to look in the mirror and really decide whether I was happy with who was looking back at me...

So let's pause here and say this out loud together:

Self-care DOES NOT EQUAL self-indulgence.

Rest is not you being lazy.

Boundaries are not a sign of you being rude.

Slowing down is not quitting.

Asking for help is not a weakness.

Choosing yourself isn't betrayal; it is self-loyalty in action.

The Guilt is Real...But So Is the Programming

You don't feel guilty for taking care of yourself because you're broken; you feel guilty because you were taught to.

We live in a world—especially in certain cultures, faith traditions, and generational cycles—that glorifies not only exhaustion, but **sacrifice**. That tells us being tired is a badge of honor. That the best kind of love is selfless, even to the point of self-erasure.

Let me tell you something:

Sacrificing your well-being for others is not sustainable!!!

Ensuring everyone else's happiness and comfort is not a life plan.

Burnout is not a personality trait.

If you were taught that your job is to suffer quietly, show up endlessly, and only rest once everything is handled, this chapter is your permission slip to start unlearning that.

Especially If You're a Caregiver...

This one is especially for the caregivers. The parents. The helpers. The eldest children. The first-generation leaders. The community builders. The ones who carry *everyone* else.

Let's be honest: most of the people who struggle to rest or receive are the ones who have been everyone's emergency contact for years.

And I get it.

It feels wrong to care for yourself when other people need you.

It feels risky to stop moving because everything you carry might collapse.

It feels unnatural to ask, "What do I need?" when you've been trained to scan the room for what everyone else is missing.

But listen—**you can't hold up everyone else while you're sinking.**

Choosing care isn't abandoning others. It's making sure you're still standing to show up again-healthy, whole, and ready.

Self-Care Isn't Something You Earn

Let's go ahead and cancel the idea that you have to "earn" rest, love, or care.

You don't earn a breath. You take one.

You don't earn time. You make it.

You don't earn self-care. You need it to live.

When we treat care as a reward for productivity, we trap ourselves in a cycle of depletion.

It sounds like:

- "Once I finish this, then I'll rest."

- "I'll relax when everyone else is okay."

- "I'll eat when I have time."

- "I'll ask for help when I really need it."

But the reality is, by the time you "deserve" it, it's often already too late.

So I'm asking you: what would it look like to stop waiting?

What if you gave yourself care *because you're human*—not because you checked all the boxes?

Using the C.A.R.E. Tool to Break the Shame Cycle

Let's bring the C.A.R.E. Tool into this moment—because this is exactly where it shines.

When the shame creeps in, when the guilt rises, when you feel like you have to earn your own humanity—go back to this framework:

C – Clarity

Ask: *Where is this guilt coming from? Whose voice is this?*

Sometimes guilt isn't a signal that you've done something wrong—it's a sign you're breaking a generational pattern.

A – Activity

Check in with your body. Are you pushing past fatigue? Are you ignoring signals of stress or pain? What would movement or stillness look like if it came from love, not punishment?

R – Resilience

Name the emotion. Are you sad? Overwhelmed? Angry that you even have to defend your rest? Let it out. Let it be. Resilience starts with emotional honesty.

E – Engagement

Who supports your healing? Who reminds you that you matter outside of your productivity? Who models rest as a right, not a reward? Seek them out. Or be that person for yourself.

The C.A.R.E. Tool isn't just about managing burnout. It's how you *rewrite your relationship with care entirely.*

You're Allowed to Be the Main Character in Your Life

This one might ruffle some feathers—but I need you to hear it.

You don't have to be the sidekick in everyone else's story.

You are allowed to center yourself.

You're allowed to say:

- "I need time or space."

- "I'm not available for that right now."

- "I'm choosing me today."

And if that upsets someone? That's information. Not your emergency.

The people who love you *want* you whole. And the ones who only love you when you're overextending? They'll fall away when you stop performing exhaustion as proof of your worth.

Truth Bomb Reminder

"Resting doesn't make you weak. It makes you ready."

Ready to show up with intention.

Ready to stop performing and start living.

Ready to break the cycle that says you have to be tired to be worthy.

Reflection Prompts

- What messages did I receive growing up about rest, sacrifice, and worth?

- Where does guilt show up when I try to care for myself?

- What would it look like to rest *bef*ore I'm completely depleted?

Final Thought – Oxygen Mask Moment

This is your turning point. Not a dramatic one, but a real, quiet, powerful one.

This is where you stop calling your own needs "too much."

This is where you stop apologizing for being human.

This is where you stop waiting for rest to feel deserved.

You don't owe anyone an explanation for taking care of yourself. Full stop.

Chapter Seven
Self-Care Is Maintenance, Not Rescue

"Almost everything will work again if you unplug it for a few minutes. Even you." – Anne Lamott

---

There's something I need you to hear right now—especially if you've been treating self-care like a fire extinguisher behind glass:

Self-care is not just what you do after everything falls apart.

It's how you keep from falling apart in the first place by putting yourself first.

We don't brush our teeth only after we get a cavity (although we do spend more time on them the day we go to the dentist). We don't wait until we're dehydrated to drink water (well... most of the time). We don't put gas in a car only when it's completely empty (again, I am a work in progress.)

So why do we treat self-care like a last resort instead of regular maintenance?

Because that's what we've been taught. We're conditioned to keep pushing through until the crash comes. Until the shutdown. Until the tears in the car, the fight with our partner, the anxiety attack in the grocery store parking lot (I have experienced all of the above).

But **you deserve more than rescue-mode living**. You deserve maintenance-mode loving. And it starts with understanding the difference between **reactive** and **proactive** care.

Reactive Self-Care: The Emergency Reset

We've all been there. In fact, I lived here for years before my breakdown.

You ignore the signs: the tension headaches, the irritability, the bone-deep fatigue. You push through the skipped meals, the sleepless nights, the people-pleasing, the inbox piling up. You said "yes" until you couldn't anymore.

Then it hits.

The wall. The meltdown. The moment you cancel everything, lock the door, shut the blinds, and crumble. That's **reactive self-care**—and it's necessary, sometimes. I've done it more times than I can count. We all have.

There is no shame in reactive care. Sometimes it's the only thing that reminds us we're human. Sometimes it's the first breath we take after drowning in expectations.

But we can't live our lives waiting for the next collapse.

We weren't built to constantly break and rebuild.

Proactive Self-Care: The Sustainable Strategy

Here's the shift: **what if self-care became the** way **we live, not just the**

way we recover?

What if it wasn't a big dramatic event, but a quiet series of micro-decisions?

Proactive self-care looks like:

- Saying "no" before you're resentful of the person, place, or thing

- Protecting your bedtime like your peace depends on it (because it does)

- Taking breaks before the burnout hits

- Setting boundaries when things are going well—not just when you're desperate

- Scheduling joy like you schedule meetings

- Checking in with yourself *before* you check out

Proactive care is powerful because it doesn't wait for a crisis.

It honors your energy in advance. It trusts that you're worthy of care every day, not just on the edge of collapse.

Self-Care Is Soul Hygiene

Here's the metaphor I love: self-care is like brushing your teeth.

You don't skip it for days and then scrub for four hours straight once your gums hurt.

You brush every day, maybe not perfectly, maybe not always at the same time, but you keep up with it because you know it's necessary.

Self-care is hygiene for your soul. It's how you stay emotionally clear. Mentally grounded. Physically aware. Spiritually anchored.

You don't need a crisis to justify it.

You just need to believe you're worth that kind of consistency.

How the C.A.R.E. Tool Supports Maintenance Over Rescue

This is where the **C.A.R.E. Tool** comes in like the ultimate check-in system—not just for when you crash, but for staying ahead of the burnout.

Let's break it down:

C – Clarity

Proactive clarity means checking in with your mind daily, not waiting until you're overwhelmed. Ask: *Where's my mental clutter building up? What can I release today?*

Mind-dumps, screen breaks, and mental "decluttering" help you stay ahead of spiraling thoughts.

A – Activity

Are you moving your body in ways that fuel it—not punish it?

Are you stretching, resting, breathing?

Proactive activity is about building a *rhythm that honors your nervous system*, not just reacts to it when you're fried.

R – Resilience

Emotional maintenance looks like regular check-ins, naming your feelings, and giving them safe outlets—before they erupt.

This might be journaling, therapy, music, movement, or just sitting in silence and letting your feelings *be*.

E – Engagement

Are you making time for connection *before* loneliness takes root?

Are you creating spiritual or social rituals that fill your cup?

Proactive engagement means weaving connection into your week, not waiting until you feel isolated and disconnected.

The C.A.R.E. Tool isn't a fix. It's a foundation.

It's how we practice sustainable self-care, one choice at a time.

The Problem With "All or Nothing" Self-Care

One of the reasons we default to reactive care is because we think anything less than a full day off or a week-long vacation doesn't count.

We wait for the "right time." The big window. The blank space on the calendar that never comes.

But maintenance-mode care *doesn't need a full reset*. It just needs intention.

It sounds like:

- "I have five minutes—I'm going to stretch."

- "I'm overwhelmed—I'll mind-dump for three minutes before my next call."

- "I'm lonely—I'll send one voice note to someone who makes me feel safe."

- "I'm tired—I'll eat something nourishing instead of skipping the meal entirely."

Self-care doesn't need to be dramatic.

It just needs to be done. Consistently. Kindly. Intentionally.

Real Talk Reminder

> **"Resting doesn't make you weak.**
> **It makes you intentional."**
> Maintenance isn't glamorous, but it's powerful.

Because the truth is, real power isn't in the comeback. It's in the stability that keeps you from breaking down in the first place.

Reflection Prompts

- Do I usually practice self-care reactively or proactively?

- What are three micro-boundaries I can put in place this week to prevent burnout?

- What small, repeatable acts of care can I make part of my daily rhythm?

Final Thought – Oxygen Mask Moment

If you're only reaching for care when things are falling apart, you're not doing it wrong. You're doing it the way most of us were taught.

But now?

You get to rewrite that story.

You get to build a version of care that's sustainable. Steady. Rooted.

You get to choose maintenance over mayhem.

Support over scramble.

Clarity, Activity, Resilience, and Engagement—on purpose, not just in panic.

You don't have to wait until you're gasping for air to put your oxygen mask on.

Put it on now. Breathe. And stay ready.

Chapter Eight
The Four Domains of Self-Care

"The challenge is not to be perfect—it is to be whole."
- Jane Fonda

I thought I was doing self-care. I really did.

A year ago, I had a particularly rough stretch. You know the kind—when everything on the outside looks manageable, but inside you're running on fumes. I was saying yes to ALL the things. I was being "productive," showing up for everyone, ticking off boxes, looking like I had it together. The usual.

I remember one week specifically. I had five different commitments in one day. I hadn't eaten a full meal sitting down in almost a week. I was eating mini pancakes and chugging Iced Lavender Oat Matchas (half-sweet, light ice, non-dairy cold foam) like it was my only sense of proper hydration and sustenance. One day, I caught myself crying in my car on the way home (I hate crying; it makes me feel weak—I am a work in progress). Not a breakdown. Not a dramatic scene. Just this quiet, exhausted drip of emotion—like my body had given up asking nicely and was now just leaking sadness wherever it could find a crack.

I remember thinking, But I've been doing self-care... haven't I?

I'd gotten my nails done. I'd posted an inspirational quote. I'd gotten my weekly 90-minute massage. I had gone to my weekly therapy session.

But clearly, none of that touched the deep, unmet needs that were silently screaming at me for attention.

That was the moment I realized I had been treating self-care like a surface fix. Don't get me wrong—all those things felt fantastic in the moment, but what I really needed was a full-body, full-soul tune-up.

Self-Care Isn't Just One Thing. It's Everything.

Self-care isn't one lane. It's a whole freaking intersection. And if we're only tending to one realm of our being—say, the physical—while ignoring the emotional, the mental, or the relational... we stay out of balance.

We might look okay on the outside. But we know when something's off.

The fog. The fatigue. The edge of irritation. The emptiness in spaces that used to bring joy. It shows up. Sometimes subtly, sometimes like a freight train.

So let's break this down the way it was meant to be lived: as a **whole-self practice**.

In this chapter, we're going to reconnect with the **four domains of self-care** using the **C.A.R.E. Tool**—Clarity, Activity, Resilience, and Engagement. These aren't separate categories. They're integrated parts of what makes you...you.

When one is depleted, the others feel it. When one is nurtured, the others benefit.

It's all connected.

Let's look at each domain. Not with perfection, but with compassion.

Clarity | *Mental Self-Care*

This is the space where we protect our minds from drowning in all of the noise.

For me, mental overload shows up like an internal pressure cooker. I stopped sleeping well. I forget simple things (and it's not just because of my ADHD). My brain gets loud but unproductive—full of spirals, to-do lists, and imagined conversations that haven't even happened yet.

Mental self-care through the Clarity lens is about:

- Saying no to what clouds your thinking—even if it's "small"

- Scheduling quiet like it's sacred (because honestly, it is)

- Turning off notifications, even for an hour, to give your brain peace

- Journaling, mind-dumping, or simply sitting in stillness for five minutes without a single goal

Clarity isn't the absence of thoughts. It's the practice of giving your mind room to exhale.

You don't need to clear your calendar to do it. You just need to create space within yourself.

Activity | *Physical Self-Care*

This isn't about boot camps or juice cleanses (neither will you ever find me doing...okay, maybe I did a juice cleanse once for like a solid 2 days).

It's about how we **listen to our body** instead of ignoring, punishing, or pushing it.

There was a time I used to interpret exhaustion as weakness. I'd push through. Grind harder. Then wonder why I got sick so often or felt disconnected from my own body.

Physical self-care through the Activity lens is about:

- Checking in: *Am I tired? Am I hungry? Am I tensing my body right now?*

- Moving your body in ways that feel like celebration, not punishment

- Nourishing yourself without shame

- Sleeping like it's part of your healing (because it is)

And sometimes? Physical self-care is doing nothing.

It's lying down. Drinking water. Saying, "I'll get to that to-morrow," and actually meaning it.

Resilience | *Emotional Self-Care*

I know what it feels like to stuff emotions down so far you almost forget they're there—until they burst out side-ways.

You think you're fine until someone cuts you off in traf-fic and you're screaming at them (okay, but to be fair, the QEW evokes a lot of emotions from a lot of people), not because of them, but because your body has finally hit capacity.

Resilience isn't about "bouncing back."

It's about allowing yourself to *feel fully* so you don't go numb.

Emotional self-care through the Resilience lens looks like:

- Letting yourself cry without needing to explain it

- Getting angry in safe spaces, instead of bottling it up

- Naming your feelings, even if they feel inconvenient

- Learning your emotional triggers—and tending to the wounds they came from

Sometimes self-care is messy. It's tears on a pillow. It's voice notes to your best friend that start with "I don't even know why I'm so upset..." It's music that understands you before you understand yourself (This is Coldplay for me).

It's giving your heart a safe place to land.

Engagement | *Relational Self-Care*

This one is layered.

Because many of us were raised to think that self-care is solo work. And yes, some of it is. But we were never meant to heal alone. Connection is care.

And when we've been burned, overextended, or taught to be "the strong one," letting people in can feel risky.

Relational self-care through the Engagement lens means:

- Unplugging from relationships that leave you drained, anxious, or small (this is friendships, family members, co-workers)

- Asking for help without apologizing for it

- Letting people know when you're not okay—without needing to perform okay-ness first

- Building and maintaining relationships that pour into you, not just pull from you (read this one again)

You don't need a huge circle. You need people who get it. People who let you take your mask off. People who hold space for you when you fall apart and don't demand you fix it by morning.

And if you're still finding those people? That's okay too. Start with being one for *yourself.*

Self-Care That Grows With You

The beauty of these four realms is that they grow with you. What self-care looks like at your busiest season will not be the same as what it looks like when you're thriving. And that's okay.

The key is noticing where you're undernourished, and offering yourself what you need now—not what you *used to* need, or what looks good on Instagram.

Check in with yourself:

- Is my mind racing? → I need **Clarity**

- Is my body tired? → I need **Activity** that restores me

- Is my heart heavy? → I need **Resilience** to feel and process

- Am I feeling alone? → I need **Engagement**, safe and soft

The more we practice this check-in, the more natural it becomes.

Reflection Prompts

"What does self-care look like when I'm thriving?

What does it look like when I'm just surviving?"

This is one of the most powerful reflections you can carry with you.

Let it guide your rhythms. Let it hold up a mirror. Let it remind you that even in survival mode, *you still deserve care.*

Final Thought – Oxygen Mask Moment

Self-care isn't a reward.

It's a rhythm.

A return.

A rescue you don't have to wait for.

Whether you're thriving, surviving, or somewhere in between—you are worth the kind of care that meets you fully. Mentally. Physically. Emotionally. Relationally.

You don't have to do it all at once.

Just begin with one breath, one check-in, one moment of truth.

You are not too far gone.

You are not too broken.

You are still in there—and you are worth the rescue *before* the emergency.

Chapter Nine
Self-Care in Real Life
(Not Just on Sundays)

"And now that you don't have to be perfect, you can be good."
– John Steinbeck

I remember one Thursday afternoon when I closed my laptop mid-sentence and cried.

It wasn't even a bad day. Nothing had "happened." No major conflict, no external chaos. But inside? I was literally running on empty.

Emails were piling up. Deadlines were breathing down my neck. I hadn't eaten anything besides a fruit snack, some strawberries, and an Earl Grey tea. My shoulders were tight, my chest was heavy, and my brain was buzzing—but not with anything helpful. Just static. Just noise.

I looked around the room, then at the life clutter in the corner, and whispered to myself, "I need to stop pretending I'm fine."

So I closed the laptop.

Left the dishes in the sink.

Curled up in bed.

And took a nap.

And for the first time that week. I breathed.

No bubble bath. No fancy planner. Just a nap.

And it felt radical.

Because sometimes the most powerful self-care you can give yourself isn't glamorous.

It's permission. To pause. To opt out. To honor the quiet "no more" that your body whispers when your mind is still trying to push through.

The Myth of the "Self-Care Sunday" Life

We've been sold this version of self-care that only exists on slow mornings and spa days. You know the vibe: fluffy robes, clean spaces, oat milk lattes (okay, but legit, these are delicious in the most non-pretentious way), perfectly lit candles. Don't get me wrong—there's nothing wrong with that kind of softness. Sometimes that's exactly what we need.

But the truth? Most of us aren't living in that aesthetic.

We're juggling work, caregiving, family responsibilities, brain fog, burnout, and a million unspoken things in between. We don't always have the time or space to *romanti-cize* our recovery. We're just trying to make it through the week. Honestly, sometimes the day.

That's why this chapter is so important.

Because **self-care in real life doesn't wait for the perfect conditions.**

It happens in the middle of the mess. It's gritty, imperfect, awkward, and sometimes **deeply** uncomfortable.

But it's also where the most *honest* healing happens.

Real-Life Self-Care Sounds Like

- "I'm leaving this group chat because it's too much noise."

- "I'm eating a sandwich sitting on the floor because I need five minutes of peace."

- "I'm letting that call go to voicemail."

- "I'm choosing therapy over pretending."

- "I'm asking for help even though I usually don't."

- "I'm not folding this laundry tonight because my body is telling me to rest."

Let's stop pretending that self-care is something that only happens when everything else is handled.

It's how we *handle* everything else.

C.A.R.E. in the Chaos

This is where your **C.A.R.E. Tool** becomes more than a framework—it becomes a *lifeline*.

When life is full, chaotic, or just plain hard, you don't need a 10-step ritual. You need real-time access to yourself. Here's how your C.A.R.E. Tool shows up in everyday ways:

Clarity (Mental)

- Turning off your phone for an hour because your brain feels fried

- Writing down your to-dos to stop the spiraling

- Canceling plans you made when you were feeling energetic, but now you're just surviving

Activity (Physical)

- Stretching in between meetings instead of pushing through

- Choosing food that fuels you instead of skipping meals

- Napping without guilt because rest is not laziness—it's recovery

Resilience (Emotional)

- Letting yourself cry in the shower because it's the only quiet moment you've had

- Texting a friend: "I'm not okay, but I'm trying"

- Naming your burnout before it becomes a break-down

Engagement (Relational)

- Saying no to the family dinner when you're too drained to hold conversation

- Delegating tasks at work instead of being the "go-to" for everything

- Creating space from someone who keeps crossing your boundaries—even if they don't mean to

Radical Doesn't Always Look Dramatic

We often think of self-care as a grand gesture—a bold moment of reclamation. And sometimes it is. But most of the time?

It's **small, repeated acts of self-honoring.**

The things no one claps for. The moments that don't make it to your social media feed.

But those are the moments that save you. That ground you. That remind you: *you're allowed to choose yourself.*

Because guess what? No one's handing out medals for self-neglect (I feel like at one point I would have won Gold).

You won't win a prize for being the most burnt out.

You don't earn your worth by sacrificing your sanity.

You're allowed to rest before you're wrecked.

You're allowed to pause before you explode.

You're allowed to make your care a priority in the middle of a messy, real, non-aesthetic life.

Self-Care Isn't Selfish—It's Strategic

You can't wait for the world to slow down.

You can't wait for the calendar to clear.

You *can* wait forever trying to find the "right time" to care for yourself.

Or—you can start with this moment. This breath. This decision.

The laundry can wait. Your wellness can't.

The inbox will still be there. Your peace is what's urgent.

The world can adjust. Your worth is not up for negotiation.

Reflection Prompts

Think about your past week.

- What did self-care *actually* look like?

- Was it saying no?

- Was it a snack?

- Was it walking away from a tense conversation?

- Was it crying in the car and then driving home with the music up?

Whatever it was, that counts.

You don't need a perfect routine. You need permission to listen to yourself in real time.

Final Thought – Oxygen Mask Moment

Self-care is not a weekend activity.

It's not a special event.

It's not something you earn by burning yourself out first.

Self-care is a Tuesday afternoon boundary.

It's a Wednesday morning cry.

It's a Thursday nap while the dishes pile up—and the world doesn't fall apart.

That's the truth no one tells us:

You can choose you, and the world will keep spinning.

So go ahead. Pause. Rest. Speak up. Unplug.

Let self-care live in the messy, the mundane, the middle of your real life.

Not just on Sundays.

Chapter Ten
Self-Care Is a Boundary,
a Practice, and a Birthright

"You cannot thrive in a system that celebrates your self-abandonment. Choose you. Every time." – Unknown

---

I used to think boundaries meant rejection.

I thought they meant cutting people off. Hurting feelings. Creating distance where I was supposed to be creating connection.

What I didn't realize was that **the only connection I was keeping intact was the one between me and my burn-out.** I wasn't choosing people. I was choosing pleasing people. I wasn't being kind. I was being complicit in my own depletion.

One of the hardest boundaries I've ever had to set wasn't with someone else.

It was with me.

With the version of me that thought I had to earn my rest.

With the voice in my head that said, "Just one more thing before you stop."

With the identity I'd built around being strong, capable, and endlessly available.

That version of me wasn't bad. She was just tired. She was scared. She was shaped by a world that celebrated her hustle but never saw her exhaustion.

And eventually, she realized something: **you can't heal in a system that benefits from your self-neglect.**

Self-Care Is a Boundary

Not a brick wall. Not a punishment. Not a tantrum.

A *boundary* is a loving limit. A sacred pause. A declaration of worth.

It sounds like:

- "That doesn't work for me."

- "I'm not available for that anymore."

- "I need space, and I'm allowed to take it."

- "I'm not abandoning you—I'm honoring me."

Setting boundaries was one of the hardest emotional muscles I had to build. Because for a long time, I was convinced that my availability equaled my value. I was afraid of coming off rude or entitled, not a team player, not a good partner, mother, daughter, or friend.

But here's the truth no one told me:

The most loving thing you can do for yourself and others is to know your limits and protect your peace.

Every yes that drains you becomes a no to yourself.

And friend, you deserve your own yes.

Self-Care Is a Practice

We love the idea of one-time transformations. The big moment. The dramatic decision.

But in real life? Self-care is more like taking a shower. Daily. Quiet. Sometimes boring. But absolutely vital.

It's a practice.

- A practice of returning to yourself over and over, especially when you stray.

- A practice of noticing when your old patterns are creeping back in.

- A practice of trying again—without shame—when you slip.

Some days, my practice looks like a full pause: journaling, canceling plans, drinking soda water like it's medicine. Other days, it's one deep breath between meetings and a silent reminder: You're doing enough. You're allowed to rest.

Self-care isn't performative.

It's not curated.

It doesn't always come with candles or captions.

It's a quiet, persistent act of remembering yourself.

Of choosing softness over striving.

Of giving yourself what you've been giving everyone else.

Over time, this practice becomes muscle memory. And one day, you catch yourself saying "no" without guilt. Catching your burnout before it brews. Speaking your needs in real-time. And you realize—you're not just surviving anymore. You're living aligned.

Self-Care Is a Birthright

This might be the most important thing I've ever written in this book, so let me say it LOUDY, BOLDY, AND CLEARLY:

You do not have to earn your own care.

Not with how productive you've been.

Not with how selfless you've acted.

Not with how well you've managed to keep it all together.

You deserve rest because you exist.

You deserve peace because you are human.

You deserve softness, safety, space, and sustenance, because you were born.

This is not a reward. This is your birthright.

It is not a luxury. It is not indulgent. It is not something reserved for when the kids are asleep, the emails are answered, the house is clean, and you've crossed some invisible finish line.

If you're breathing, you are worthy.

If you're waking up each day and trying, you are worthy.

If you are burned out and unsure how to begin again— you are still worthy.

You don't have to prove your pain for it to be valid.

You don't have to justify your need for care.

The moment you decide that *you matter* is the moment self-care becomes non-negotiable.

What This Looks Like in Real Life

Let me give you a few snapshots of what this shift actually looks like—because theory is great, but this book is about real life.

- You say "no" to a meeting and don't explain why.
- You take a nap with a sink full of dishes and choose rest anyway.
- You unfollow someone who triggers your comparison spiral.

- You choose therapy over being the strong friend every single time.

- You don't respond right away. To the texts. To the emails. To the pressure.

- You speak a truth you've been swallowing for years—and survive the silence that follows.

- You let go of the version of you that coped through chaos—and welcome the version that craves peace.

Each of those is a form of self-care. Each is a moment of returning home to yourself.

REFLECTION PROMPT

> Ask Yourself: "What does it mean for me to belong to myself first?"

This question cracked me ALL THE WAY open.

Because I had belonged to other people for so long—belonged to their opinions, their expectations, their comfort. I was so good at being what everyone needed me to be, I forgot who I actually was.

Belonging to yourself doesn't mean you reject others.

It means you stop rejecting *you* (read that again).

It means you sit with your full self—your desires, your limits, your grief, your softness—and say:

You're allowed. You're safe here.
You don't need to disappear to be loved.

Final Thought – Oxygen Mask Moment

You are not selfish for needing care.

You are not dramatic for needing space.

You are not weak for needing help.

You are not "being extra" for telling the truth of your needs.

You cannot thrive in a system that celebrates your self-abandonment.

So, don't wait for that system to validate your worth.

Don't wait for burnout to give you permission to pause.

Don't wait for a breakdown to finally say, "Enough."

Say it now.

Choose yourself now.

Even when it disappoints others.

Even when it's scary.

Even when you don't know what comes next.

Because self-care isn't just a boundary or a break.

It's your return.

To your body.

To your values.

To your inner voice that always knew what you needed—long before the world told you to forget.

Section Three
Not Enough Time in the Day?

Practical, No-Cost Self-Care Ideas to Make Your Day Work for You

If you've made it this far, first—take a deep breath. Seriously. Pause for a moment and acknowledge how far you've come in this journey. You've started to challenge some deeply ingrained beliefs about burnout, self-worth, and the myth of "doing it all."

But let's be real: even with all this insight, there's still one narrative that's especially hard to shake. One that creeps into your calendar, your nervous system, and your subconscious:

"There's just not enough time."

Section Three is here to bust that myth—and give you tools to reclaim your time, your energy, and your boundaries without needing a week off, a retreat, or a new life altogether.

This section isn't about time management. It's about time ownership.

And we start right here—with the illusion that you don't have enough.

Chapter Eleven
The Illusion of Time Scarcity

"The key to time management is to see the value of every moment." – Bryant McGill

I thought I had a time problem. But I had a boundary problem.

There was a season of my life that now feels like a fever dream. I was newly married, working four jobs, and going to school full-time. Most nights I ran on two to three hours of sleep. Weekends were for catching up—not on rest, but on everything I hadn't gotten to Monday through Friday.

People would ask, "How do you do it all?"

I'd smile, hide behind humor, and say something like, "With wine and Jesus."

But on the inside? I was unraveling.

At the time, I honestly believed I was just bad at managing my schedule. If I could just get more organized, if I could just be more efficient, I'd finally catch up.

But no amount of color-coded planners, alarms, or to-do lists could fix what was actually broken:

I wasn't overbooked.

I was **overextended**.

And I didn't have a time issue.

I had a **capacity issue**.

I was trying to do the work of five people, meet the emotional needs of everyone around me, pursue success at all costs, and somehow still show up in my marriage as a loving, present partner.

There was no "hack" for that.

There was no productivity app that could save me (I tried a lot of them).

Because what I needed wasn't more time—it was permission to live within mine.

The Time Scarcity Lie

Let's get this out of the way first:

Time scarcity is real.

But not in the way we're taught to think.

The hours in a day are limited. That's true. But the belief that we're supposed to do everything, be everything, fix everything, and still find time for joy, rest, and reflection?

That's not a time issue.

That's an expectation issue.

When you've been conditioned to associate worth with output, it's no wonder you feel like there's never enough time. You're not just trying to keep up—you're trying to prove you deserve to pause.

And that's where the burnout cycle sneaks in:

- You overcommit because you feel guilty saying no.

- You start running on fumes.

- You push harder because "there's no time to rest."

- You finally crash—and blame it on poor time management.

- Rinse. Repeat.

But here's the truth most people won't say out loud:

Time isn't the problem. The pace is.

And if we don't start examining the *pace* we're living at, no amount of scheduling will save us from collapse.

Time Isn't Just a Clock—It's Capacity

You and I have the same 24 hours as everyone else.

But not everyone has the same:

- Workplace Expectations

- Mental bandwidth

- Physical energy

- Support system

- Health needs

- Social demands

We have to stop pretending that time exists in a vacuum.

A single mom working two jobs doesn't have the same 24 hours as someone with flexible work-from-home options and access to childcare.

A person living with chronic pain doesn't have the same energy window as someone who wakes up feeling fully rested.

Someone navigating trauma or grief or ADHD or high-functioning anxiety isn't starting from the same baseline of focus or capacity.

So no, you're not lazy. You're not undisciplined. You're not bad at time management.

You're human.

And your time has to be built around your reality, not your shame.

What Time Stewardship Actually Looks Like

Instead of asking: *How can I do more in less time?*

Ask: *What actually deserves my energy?*

Self-care in this context means redefining how you show up inside your time—not just how much of it you use.

Let's apply the **C.A.R.E. Tool** here:

Clarity (Mental)

- Identify your "shoulds" versus your actual priorities
- Mind-dump your mental load so your brain has space
- Choose one micro-priority per day to feel accomplished without overloading

Activity (Physical)

- Schedule rest like it matters—because it does
- Move your body based on energy, not guilt
- Protect your sleep like it's a sacred appointment

Resilience (Emotional)

- Recognize the emotional labor hiding in your day
- Say no without apology—your bandwidth is not endless
- Acknowledge that doing less can sometimes be the brave thing

Engagement (Relational)

- Reevaluate where your time leaks are (toxic group chats, guilt-driven hangouts)

- Build in time for connection that fuels you—not drains you

- Be honest when you're maxed out—let people see your humanity

Time Is Not Just a Resource. It's a Reflection.

How you use your time tells a story.

Is it a story of survival?

Of over-functioning?

Of keeping up appearances?

Or is it becoming a story of alignment?

When you begin to tell yourself the truth—that your time is finite, that your energy is sacred, that your worth is not measured by your busyness—you stop chasing balance and start reclaiming **ownership.**

You don't need more hours. You need more honesty.

REFLECTION PROMPTS

Let's Pause Here

Take a second and reflect:

- When was the last time you felt time-rich instead of time-starved?

- What are you spending time on that doesn't align with your values?

- Who or what has been writing your time story for you?

And most importantly:

> What would it look like to treat your time like it belongs to you?

FINAL THOUGHT – The Oxygen Mask Moment

This isn't about perfection. This is about permission.

Permission to slow down.

Permission to choose less.

Permission to stop believing that your value is tied to your productivity.

You don't need to earn your time.

You just need to honor it.

Because when your oxygen mask is on, time stops being something you chase—and starts being something that works with you.

Chapter Twelve
The Time Trap — Busy vs. Productive

"Rest doesn't steal time; it creates it. When you rest, you reset." – Unknown

I used to wear "busy" like a badge.

There was a time in my life when, if someone asked how I was doing, I'd instinctively reply, "Busy, but good!" or "I'm good, just living the dream!"

Even when I wasn't good. Even when I was quietly unraveling.

I confused exhaustion with importance. I believed that my packed schedule proved my ambition, that my constant motion confirmed my resilience. In truth? I was terrified that if I ever stopped, even for a second, everything would fall apart—including me.

I remember one day in particular: I had back-to-back meetings, a paper due for school, three different job shifts in a 36-hour window, and barely enough time to eat. I was beyond tired—I was fried. But instead of canceling or delegating, I pushed harder. I told myself, "This is just the grind. You'll rest later."

Spoiler alert: later never came.

What did come was a meltdown in the break room of one of my jobs, when my supervisor gently asked if I was okay. I burst into tears, not because of anything she said—but because the question caught me off guard. It reminded me that I hadn't actually checked in with myself in weeks.

I wasn't okay.

I was **overbooked, overfunctioning, and emotionally bankrupt.**

That day marked the beginning of my awareness around the difference between being busy and being productive. Because up until then, I had been **busy** nonstop—but I hadn't actually been moving forward.

Busy Is a Feeling. Productive Is an Outcome.

Let's get this straight: Busy and productive are not the same thing.

We confuse the two because, let's face it, being busy feels like you're doing something important. When you're busy, your calendar is full, your notifications are nonstop, your body is in motion. It's loud. It's visible. People notice.

Productivity, on the other hand, is quiet. It's intentional. It's not always flashy or externally validated. Sometimes it means doing less, not more.

Here's the distinction:

Busy	Productive
Reactive	Intentional
Overcommitted	Prioritized
Chaotic multitasking	Focused execution
Emotionally draining	Emotionally sustainable
Fueled by guilt or fear	Fueled by clarity and alignment
Measured by time and effort	Measured by results and impact

Why We Keep Ourselves Busy

Let's dig into the why behind the constant hustle. If you're anything like me, you've probably found yourself doing the absolute most at times you should have been doing the very least.

Here's why that happens:

1. Fear of Falling Behind

We live in a culture obsessed with speed. If you're not constantly doing something, someone else is—right? And they'll get ahead. So we move fast, say yes too often, and cram our days with activity because we're afraid of what it means to slow down.

But here's the truth: You can't fall behind on a path that's uniquely yours. Your journey isn't a race. It's a rhythm.

2. Guilt for Resting

This is a big one. Especially for caregivers, high achievers, and people raised in environments where value was tied to sacrifice. Rest can feel like slacking. Pausing can feel selfish. So instead of giving ourselves permission to be still, we keep moving to silence the shame.

3. Chasing Worth Through Work

For years, I believed that if I stayed busy enough, no one could call me lazy. That if I kept showing up for everyone, I'd prove I was dependable. Underneath all of that? A deep fear of being seen as not enough.

If any of this resonates with you, you're not alone. But you *are* allowed to challenge it.

Rewriting the Narrative

We've been fed the idea that being busy means we matter. That burnout is a byproduct of ambition. That if we just try harder, we'll finally feel fulfilled.

But this is what I've learned: **Being busy often masks the parts of us that feel unseen, unworthy, or unsafe when still.**

It's not laziness we're fighting. It's the discomfort of being with ourselves.

So, what if we redefined the narrative?

Old Script: "If I'm not busy, I'm not valuable."

New Truth: "My value is in who I am—not in how much I do."

Old Script: "Rest is a waste of time."

New Truth: "Rest doesn't steal time. It restores it."

Old Script: "Productivity means constant motion."

New Truth: "Productivity is progress—not just activity."

Applying the C.A.R.E. Tool: Busy vs. Productive

Here's how you can filter your daily habits through the C.A.R.E. lens to shift from busy to aligned:

Clarity (Mental)

Ask: "Is this task meaningful, or just filling space?"

- Use mind-dumps to get honest about what's essential vs. urgent.

- Create buffer time between tasks to reduce mental whiplash.

Activity (Physical)

- Honor your body's signals. Are you fatigued or just stimulated?

- Build in recovery time. Real productivity includes *pause points.*

- Don't use movement or busyness as avoidance—be intentional.

Resilience (Emotional)

- Check in with your *why*. Are you doing this to avoid a feeling?

- Allow rest without emotional debt. You don't owe anyone your exhaustion.

- Journal about where guilt shows up around slowing down.

Engagement (Relational)

- Be honest when your schedule is full—don't over-promise to protect peace.

- Surround yourself with people who value *your well-being*, not just your output.

- Let go of urgency culture—it's not your responsibility to respond instantly.

REFLECTION PROMPTS

Sometimes we can't just stop everything. Life is real, responsibilities are real, bills are real. But we *can* interrupt the busy loop with small shifts.

Try these:

- **Daily capacity check-ins:** Ask, "What do I actually have space for today?"

- **One-task prioritizing:** If nothing else gets done, what one thing will move me forward?

- **Scheduled stillness:** When can I schedule five minutes of doing nothing?

- **Delete a "should":** What day can I choose one task or commitment I've been doing out of guilt, and let it go?

- **Two-column list:** Create your own "Must Do" vs. "Might Do." Give yourself permission not to be superhuman.

FINAL THOUGHT – The Oxygen Mask Moment

You don't have to prove your worth through motion.

You are not lazy for needing less.

You are not failing if your calendar isn't bursting at the seams.

And you are allowed to rest—not just at night, but in the middle of the day, the week, your life.

Rest isn't the opposite of productivity.

It's the foundation of it.

You can leave the busy badge behind.

You can choose presence over pressure.

You can let your value be rooted in your being—not your busyness.

And you can give yourself the gift of time—not by having more of it, but by choosing to live within it.

Chapter Thirteen
Free (But Powerful) Ways to Create More Time

"The only reason for time is so that everything doesn't happen at once." – Albert Einstein

---

There was a time when even 10 minutes felt like a luxury.

I remember sitting in my car between back-to-back obligations—text messages buzzing, emails unanswered, a to-do list growing like a weed—and I thought to myself: *I just need a second to breathe.* But instead of breathing, I checked my phone. I answered two emails. I made a mental grocery list. I filled the space instead of feeling it.

What I needed wasn't more doing.

It was *undoing.*

I didn't need to solve anything in that moment.

I just needed to **be still.** But I honestly didn't know how.

Because when your life is scheduled down to the minute, rest doesn't feel like restoration—it feels like rebellion. Even to this day, when some people look at my phone calendar, they tell me it causes them instant anxiety.

This chapter is about reclaiming those moments.

Not in hours, but in intentional pockets. Not through escape, but through empowerment.

We're going to talk about how you can create time without changing your whole life. Because the truth is, you don't need more time—you need to be in your time differently.

The 10-Minute Reset

You don't need an hour-long yoga class or a full day off to reset your nervous system.

What you need is intentional pause.

A 10-minute reset is *not*:

- Scrolling Instagram until your thumb goes numb

- Mindlessly clearing out emails

- Folding laundry while on a conference call

Those things might keep you busy, but they don't give you back to yourself.

A real 10-minute reset is about creating a break in the pattern. It's where you consciously choose to stop reacting and start regulating.

Why 10 Minutes Works

You can do anything for 10 minutes. That's why it's powerful. It's long enough to shift your energy—but short enough that your brain doesn't resist it as "too much."

This is what I call **time-liberating, not time-consuming** self-care.

Here are a few reset ideas that work with real life:

- **Deep Breathing:** 4 counts in, 7 counts hold, 8 counts out. Repeat 5 times.

- **Gentle Stretching:** Neck rolls, shoulder shrugs, wrist circles—especially if you've been hunched over a screen.

- **Step Outside:** Fresh air isn't a luxury. It's a nervous system reboot.

- **Close Your Eyes:** Not to nap. Just to rest your senses and bring your attention inward.

- **Music Reset:** One song. Eyes closed. Let the rhythm ground you.

- **Journaling Prompt:** "What am I feeling right now?" or "What do I need in this moment?"

- **Prayer or Spiritual Connection:** Praying out loud to God or connecting spiritually in whatever way you believe in.

- **Micro-Meditation:** Set a timer for 3–5 minutes. Focus on your breath or a mantra like *I return to myself.*

10 minutes. That's it. But when done consistently, this becomes your power source, not a pause button.

The Power of Saying "No"

Let's get something straight: No is a complete sentence. Full stop.

We often look for time in our calendars, our alarms, our planners. But one of the most liberating time strategies? **Saying no more often—and with less guilt.**

I get it. Saying no can feel rude, selfish, or disappointing. Especially when you're used to being the dependable one. The helper. The over-functioner.

But here's the truth:

Every time you say "yes" to something that doesn't serve you, you're saying "no" to your own well-being.

What Saying "No" Actually Looks Like

- Saying no to that extra Zoom meeting that could've been an email

- Saying no to a last-minute volunteer ask because you're maxed out

- Saying no to small talk that drains you

- Saying no to "one more thing" when you're already over capacity

- Saying no to a social hangout when your soul is craving solitude

Not every "no" needs an excuse. Not every "no" needs a backstory. Some of your nos are just boundaries—and that's enough.

But What If I Feel Bad?

Ah, guilt. Our favorite toxic side dish.

Here's the thing: **Guilt doesn't mean you're doing something wrong.**

It often means you're doing something new. Especially when you've been trained to equate your worth with your availability.

But if you want more peace, more space, more energy— you're going to have to disappoint someone. And that's okay. You're allowed to be the one who finally chooses *you*.

The "Hard No" Script

Sometimes we need words we can lean on when our people-pleasing instincts kick in. So here are a few scripts to keep in your back pocket:

- "Thanks for thinking of me. I'm not able to commit right now."

- "That sounds great, but I need to protect my bandwidth this week."

- "I can't take that on and still show up well for the things already on my plate."

- "I'm learning to say no more often—and this is one of those times."

- "That's not going to work for me right now, but I appreciate you asking."

The goal isn't to say no to everything. It's to say **yes to what matters**—and clear the rest.

REFLECTION PROMPT

Look at your calendar for the next week.
Can you identify one thing you can say no to that
isn't serving you?

FINAL THOUGHT – The Oxygen Mask Moment

You don't need more time. You need fewer things that drain your time, your soul, and your energy.

You need:

- 10 minutes to come home to yourself

- 3 deep breaths before jumping into the next task

- 1 honest "no" that protects your peace

- A few pockets of unstructured time that no one else gets to fill but *you*

Productivity will never give you peace if it's built on self-neglect.

Presence will.

Clarity will.

Boundaries will.

Rest isn't a waste.

Saying no isn't rude.

And reclaiming your time isn't selfish—it's sacred.

You don't have to *earn* your pauses. You just have to *take* them.

Chapter Fourteen
Restorative Activities
That Don't Cost a Dime

"Take care of your body. It's the only place you have to live."
– Jim Rohn

I once spent $500 trying to "feel better."

One particularly rough week, I was so emotionally depleted that I convinced myself the only way to fix it was to throw money at the problem. So I booked the massage. The facial. The salt scrub. The milk bath. The full package. I sat in the spa lounge sipping cucumber water and a mimosa, trying to force calm into my body like a transaction.

On the outside, it looked like luxury.

But on the inside? I was still carrying every ounce of burnout I had walked in with.

By the end of the day, I didn't feel restored—I felt numb.

Overstimulated. Overspent. And still emotionally exhausted.

That was the moment I realized: restoration doesn't require a fancy robe or a scented candle. It doesn't need a credit card or a curated self-care aesthetic.

What I really needed was *presence.*

What I really needed was *pause.*

What I really needed... didn't cost anything at all.

Micro-Meditations: Reset in Real Time

Let's dismantle the idea that meditation requires silence, incense, and sitting cross-legged for 30 minutes. If that works for you, beautiful. But if it feels inaccessible or unrealistic, let's start smaller.

A **micro-meditation** is a tiny act of presence.

It's a pause button for your brain.

A way to break the cycle of mental overload and come back to now.

Why It Works

Your nervous system doesn't need a retreat to reset.

It just needs a signal that you're safe.

Even 60 seconds of intentional breathing can:

- Lower anxiety

- Clear mental clutter

- Center your thoughts

- Slow your heart rate

- Improve your emotional regulation

And that's something you can do anywhere, at any time.

When to Do It:

- Before opening your inbox in the morning

- In your car before going inside

- While waiting in line

- During transitions between meetings or calls

- When you catch yourself spiraling

Try This (like in the previous chapter):

- Inhale for 4 counts

- Hold for 4 counts

- Exhale for 6 counts

- Repeat 3 times

- Say (silently or aloud): *I return to myself.*

You don't have to fix everything in that moment. You just have to **stop the spin**. You just have to remember you're allowed to come back to yourself.

Power Naps: Your Energy Reset Button

Let's reclaim naps. Seriously. I mean it. They are the best.

Somewhere along the line, we started believing that napping was lazy, or childish, or a sign that we weren't "tough enough." Meanwhile, we're walking around sleep-deprived, overstimulated, and emotionally fried, pretending like willpower alone will get us through.

Let me say it clearly: **naps are not indulgent.**

They are a *smart strategy.*

The Power of the 10–20 Minute Nap

A short, intentional nap can:

- Increase alertness
- Boost productivity
- Help prevent decision fatigue
- Lower stress hormones
- Improve emotional control and memory

It's not about crashing. It's about clearing.

And science backs this up—10 to 20 minutes is the sweet spot. Long enough to rest, short enough to avoid grogginess (because that's the worst).

How to Do It Well

- Set a **timer** for 15–20 minutes
- Create a calm space: a couch, a quiet corner, even the front seat of your car
- Put your phone on **Do Not Disturb**

- Before closing your eyes, try this:

Say:

"I'm not giving up. I'm rebooting. When I wake, I'll feel grounded and alert."

Even if you don't fall fully asleep, that intentional rest will serve you. Don't measure success by how deep you slept—measure it by how gently you returned to yourself.

Stretch Breaks: Move the Tension Out

Stress doesn't just live in your mind—it lives in your body.

And when we don't move it, it *stays there.* Our bodies carry what we don't express. Tension in our shoulders, tightness in our chest, stiffness in our hips... it's all communication.

This is me. All day long. I carry my stress in my body.

Stretching isn't just physical. It's an emotional release.

You don't need a workout. You need a few minutes to move what's stuck.

What It Does:

- Improves circulation

- Releases built-up tension

- Increases energy and focus

- Signals your nervous system that it's safe to relax

Easy Stretching Ideas:

1. The Wake-Up Reach

Stand up. Reach both arms toward the ceiling. Inhale deeply. Hold for 10 seconds. Exhale slowly.

2. Shoulder Roll Relief

Roll your shoulders forward 10 times. Then backward 10 times. Let your breath guide the rhythm.

3. Seated Spinal Twist

Sit tall, place one hand on the opposite knee, and gently twist. Hold. Breathe. Switch sides.

4. Chest Opener

Clasp your hands behind your back. Pull your arms straight, gently lifting your chest. Inhale into your heart space.

When to Stretch:

- After sitting too long
- During a break in the day
- While your coffee or tea brews
- While brushing your teeth
- Right before bed to release the day

Stretching isn't performance. It's presence.

It's saying: *I remember I have a body, and I choose to be in it.*

REFLECTION PROMPT

Try This: Stand up, reach for the ceiling, and stretch for 30 seconds. Close your eyes and breathe deeply.

How do you feel in your body? Write it out.

FINAL THOUGHT - Oxygen Mask Moment

You don't need a $100 massage to deserve a break.

You don't need a three-day weekend to feel restored.

You don't need a "treat" to justify basic nervous system care.

What you do need is:

- **One minute of breath**
- **One honest pause**
- **One act of coming home to yourself**

Rest isn't a detour. It's the path, and you are allowed to take it—without guilt, without waiting, without needing permission.

These tools aren't soft.

They're strong.

They are how we survive the day without abandoning ourselves.

Chapter Fifteen
The Art of Doing Nothing
(And Why It's Essential)

"Doing nothing often leads to the very best of something."
– Winnie the Pooh

I once scheduled "doing nothing"—and then couldn't figure out how to do it.

No joke. I literally put it in my calendar.

"Block: Doing absolutely nothing. No errands. No emails. No people."

It was a Tuesday afternoon. The house was quiet. I sat down on the couch with a blanket and a warm mug of tea in front of my fireplace, ready to embrace my much-needed reset.

And within five minutes, I was spiraling. Was it that my ADHD meds hadn't kicked in yet?

I thought about the dishes in the sink.

Then the unread emails.

Then the text I hadn't replied to.

Then whether this was even productive rest or if I was just being lazy.

Then whether my "doing nothing" was being done right.

I was literally stressed out about trying to relax.

It was in that moment I realized something sobering: I had completely **unlearned how to be still,** and it wasn't because I didn't know how to sit on a couch.

It was because somewhere along the way, I had tied my worth to my output.

Stillness Is Not Laziness

We live in a culture that celebrates overachievement and glorifies exhaustion.

The person who sleeps the least, hustles the most, and stays busiest is often the one we applaud. We're conditioned to believe that rest must be earned and that stillness is suspicious.

But here's the truth I had to learn the hard way:

Doing nothing is not wasting time.

Doing nothing is reclaiming time.

Rest isn't passive. It's powerful, because in those quiet, unproductive moments, your mind resets. Your nervous system rebalances. Your heart finally gets a chance to catch up with everything your body's been carrying.

And let me tell you, it's not always comfortable—but it's absolutely essential.

Unlearning the "Always-On" Mindset

Let's be honest: we are constantly on.

Even when we're technically "off," we're still *on*—on our phones, on edge, on deadlines, on call.

The "always-on" mentality is exhausting because it never lets our brain close the tab. We're running 47 mental programs in the background at all times.

We tell ourselves:

- "I'll rest when I finish everything."

- "I don't have time to slow down."

- "There's too much to do to just sit there."

But here's the catch: everything is never finished.

There will always be one more load of laundry, one more email, one more thing pulling your attention. If you wait for life to create stillness for you, you'll wait forever.

That's why you have to create the stillness yourself.

What "Doing Nothing" Actually Looks Like

Doing nothing doesn't mean zoning out on Netflix for hours or mindlessly scrolling social media (but I get it, some of those shows are made for binging).

This is about intentional stillness. It is about **moments in which nothing is required of you**—not your brain, not your body, not your emotions.

It can look like:

- Sitting on the porch and staring at the sky

- Lying on the floor and letting your body go limp

- Closing your eyes and listening to silence

- Gazing out the window with no agenda

- Sitting on the couch and letting your thoughts drift like clouds

No journaling. No breathwork. No playlist. No productivity attached.

Just **you, being with yourself**.

And the wildest part? Our brain and body will resist it at first.

Because stillness can feel scary when you've been surviving in constant motion.

But keep going. Keep softening. That resistance is your nervous system learning that **peace is safe now.**

Protecting Your Downtime Like You Protect Your Deadlines

Let me ask you something bold:

Do you guard your rest time the way you guard your meetings?

Because most of us wouldn't dare miss a work deadline. We'd reschedule sleep, meals, even bathroom breaks to meet a commitment.

But when it comes to our *downtime*? We give it away like it costs nothing.

Here's what I've learned: **if you don't protect your peace, it will be claimed by everything and everyone else.**

So what if you blocked your calendar for "Nothing Time" like you do your Zoom meetings?

What if you put up an autoresponder for your energy?

What if you said, out loud or silently:

I'm not available to be productive right now.

I'm in recovery mode.

And you actually *meant it and followed through.*

Building Stillness Into Your Week

You don't have to go off-grid or cancel everything to practice this.

Try starting with **one still moment per day**—literally five minutes.

And one "nothing hour" per week, where you give yourself full permission to unplug.

Put it in your calendar. Name it something bold:

- *Peace Hour*

- *Mental Reset Block*

- *Do Nothing, Heal Everything*

And treat it like the sacred time it is.

Because it's in the quiet that your truth shows up. It's in the space where no one's asking anything of you that your creativity returns. It's in the pause that your body gets to exhale.

Final Thought – Oxygen Mask Moment

This isn't about escaping your life. It's about creating space to return to it with intention.

Doing nothing is not a luxury. It is a **necessity** for people who carry a lot, care a lot, and give a lot.

It is a rebellion against burnout.

It is an act of resistance in a productivity-obsessed world.

It is you saying, "I deserve to exist, even when I'm not producing something."

Stillness is not empty. It's full of everything your soul has been asking for.

So the next time someone asks what you're doing, and the answer is "nothing," say it with your whole chest.

And if that someone is you? Say it louder.

Chapter Sixteen
Leveraging the Time You Have (Even When It Feels Like None)

"The key is not to prioritize what's on your schedule, but to schedule your priorities." – Stephen R Covey

---

I used to say "I don't have time" like it was a fact.

I said it when someone invited me out.

I said it when my therapist suggested journaling.

I said it when I knew I needed to rest, to eat, to stretch, to breathe.

"I would, but I just don't have time."

It felt true in the moment.

I was working. Commuting. Mothering. Helping. Showing up. Trying to be everything, to everyone, every day, all the time. But one night, sitting in bed—absolutely fried from yet another 12-hour day—I decided to scroll back through my phone's screen time report.

And that's when I saw it.

Four hours.

That day alone, I had spent **four full hours** on social media.

Now, I'm not here to shame scrolling. We all need escapes. But in that moment, I had to get radically honest with myself:

It wasn't that I didn't have time.
It was that I had **given my time away
without meaning to.**

Time Isn't "Found." It's *Created.*

Let's get something clear right now: **you are not lazy, weak, or disorganized.**

You are overwhelmed. You are exhausted. And more than likely, you are *overextended.*

The world isn't set up to help you protect your time. It's built to keep you productive, distracted, and available 24/7.

So if it feels like time is slipping through your fingers, that's not a personal failure. That's the system working exactly as it was designed.

But here's the good news: **you can disrupt it.**

You can stop waiting for time to "show up" and start **intentionally creating space** for the things that matter—including rest.

It starts with awareness.

The Power of a Time Audit

I know—tracking your time might sound like one more task. But this is not about judgment. It's about **curiosity**.

It's about asking: *Where is my energy actually going?* Because until you see it clearly, you can't change it intentionally.

Try This: The 1-Day Time Audit

I do this exercise in one of my classes with my college and high school students (but I make them do 2 days and they are marked on it). For one day, write down (or voice note) how you spend your time. All of it. From the moment you wake up until you go to bed.

Include:

- Work or school time

- Meals

- Breaks

- Screen time

- Mindless scrolls

- Commutes

- Chores

- Conversations

- Even "just five minutes" moments (they add up!)

At the end of the day, reflect:

- What surprised you?

- Where did time leak out without you noticing?

- What moments could have been reclaimed for care or clarity?

This isn't about perfection. It's about **awareness.**

You can't reclaim what you haven't recognized.

Where the Time *Actually* Goes

We often feel like we're constantly working or moving, but when we look closer, we notice:

- 15 minutes checking emails before even getting out of bed

- 30 minutes deciding what to eat because we didn't prep

- 20 minutes re-reading the same document because we're mentally fried

- 1 hour scrolling while "winding down" that didn't actually help us relax

None of those things make us bad or broken. They make us **human**.

But if we can reclaim just 10–30 minutes a day from those hidden spaces and funnel them toward intentional care? That's where the shift happens.

Multitasking = Faster Burnout

Let me call out a myth many of us live by:

"I'm good at multitasking."

Liar. No. You're good at **surviving in chaos.**

Multitasking might feel productive in the moment, but it actually makes your brain work harder. Each time you switch tasks, you create mental lag—and your nervous system pays the price.

Multitasking creates:

- Decision fatigue

- Mental clutter

- Emotional detachment from your work

- More mistakes = more time spent correcting

Instead, try **monotasking.** One thing. One focus. One breath at a time.

Even if it's just for 15 minutes:

- Eat without your phone

- Write the email without jumping tabs

- Walk without making a call

- Fold laundry while listening to music instead of working

The goal isn't to be less productive—it's to be *less scattered.*

Because scattered energy is expensive.

Hidden Pockets of Time = Hidden Gold

If you feel like your days are slammed, you're not wrong. But there are often tiny pockets of time hiding in plain sight. When I did the exercise above, it blew my mind.

So let's find yours.

Reclaimable Moments:

- The first 10 minutes after waking up

- The 5 minutes before your next meeting

- That awkward window between errands

- Your bathroom breaks (yes, seriously)

- Waiting in the car before pick-up

- Those 20 minutes when you "check one thing" and fall into the scroll

What if you used just *one* of those pockets to:

- Breathe deeply

- Stretch

- Drink water (soda water in my case)

- Write one sentence in your journal

- Step outside

- Close your eyes

That's not selfish. That's strategy.

Creating Space *On Purpose*

So how do you make space when your calendar is already full?

Start by asking:

- What can I *delegate*?

- What can I *decline*?

- What can I *defer*?

- What can I *delete* altogether?

If your plate is too full, shrinking yourself won't solve it.

You have to take something off the plate.

Your time is your most valuable, non-renewable resource. Start treating it like sacred currency.

REFLECTION Time Audit Reflection Prompt:

- What surprised me about how I used my time today?

- Where did I feel most scattered? Most grounded?

- What's one small shift I can make tomorrow to create more room for myself?

FINAL THOUGHT – The Oxygen Mask Moment

Let's stop pretending time is something you either have or don't.

Time is shaped by choices. Time is shaped by values. Time is shaped by boundaries.

You don't have to overhaul your entire life to create room for yourself. You just have to *start noticing* where your time is going—and take some of it back.

Not to be more productive.

Not to hustle harder.

But to *breathe. Reconnect. And rest.*

Chapter Seventeen
Time Is a Resource—Use It Wisely

"If you want to fly, you have to give up the things that weigh you down." – Toni Morrison

Time isn't the enemy. But ignoring it can make it feel like one.

I used to think I was bad at time management. I'd buy planners. Download apps. Try time-blocking systems. Wake up early (which I hated) to "get ahead." And still— still—I'd fall into bed at the end of the day wondering where the hours went.

But over time, I learned something important:

I didn't need more hours.

I needed to own the ones I already had.

Because the truth is, **time will never feel like "enough" until you learn to treat it like a resource you get to protect—not a monster you're constantly chasing.**

And when I stopped treating time like a punishment and started treating it like a partner, everything shifted.

Time Will Never Be Unlimited—But It's Still Yours

There's no magical future version of your life when you'll "finally have time."

There will always be dishes. Laundry. Deadlines. Family obligations. Unexpected emails. Burnt toast. Group chats. Traffic.

Time won't stretch. But your relationship to it can.

Reclaiming that relationship isn't about cramming more in—it's about getting intentional with what stays, what goes, and what finally gets prioritized.

Especially you.

Stillness Isn't Found—It's Carved

You don't need a sabbatical to find stillness.

You don't need a three-day weekend to feel joy.

You need to create moments inside the moments.

It's the **10 seconds of deep breath** before you answer a call.

It's the **3-minute lie down** on the couch between tasks.

It's the **one decision not to overbook your Saturday.**

You don't need to bulldoze your life.

You just need to carve space within it.

These "pockets" are where burnout is softened and resilience is rebuilt.

Less, But With More Intention

Let's stop pretending time management is about productivity hacks. It's not.

It's not about:

- Scheduling every hour down to the minute

- Becoming a robot of efficiency

- Hustling harder to prove your worth

Real time management—the kind that protects your well-being—is about asking:

"What do I actually want to feel today?"

"What needs to get done—and what can wait?"

"What would honoring my energy actually look like?"

It's not about doing more.

It's about doing what matters, and letting the rest go.

Try This: The Time Trade-Off Mindset

Every "yes" you say is a trade-off.

Yes to that extra meeting? That might mean no to your lunch break.

Yes to staying up late for emails? That might mean no to energy tomorrow.

Yes to one more task? That might mean no to resting.

So instead of defaulting to "yes" for everything, start asking:

"If I say yes to this, what am I saying no to?"

This isn't about guilt. It's about **alignment**. It's about making your time reflect your values—not just your obligations.

Reclaiming Sacred Time

You don't need a planner to make time sacred. You just need a boundary.

Sacred time = protected time

Time that belongs to you.

Time that doesn't require explanation.

Time that helps you remember who you are.

Try blocking off:

- A quiet morning coffee or tea—no phone, no noise
- A mid-day walk just to move your body
- An evening ritual of breathwork, prayer, or journaling
- A Friday night when you don't answer to anyone

Put it in your calendar like you would any important meeting. Because it is.

Time Is a Cycle, Not a Checklist

Some days will feel tight. Some weeks will be chaotic. That's life.

But just because your time is stretched doesn't mean you're powerless.

Every moment is a chance to return to yourself.

This isn't about perfection—it's about **returning** to intention again and again.

Because time, like self-care, is not a one-time fix. It's a rhythm.

You get to practice. You get to adjust.

You get to begin again.

REFLECTION PROMPT

> "What's one small time shift I can make to prioritize myself today?"

- A pause before responding?
- A "no" where I used to say yes?
- A moment of breath instead of multitasking?

Whatever it is—start there.

Small shifts create wide-open space.

FINAL THOUGHT – Oxygen Mask Moment

Time won't slow down for you. But you can slow down within it.

You can stop letting time push you around and start standing in your authority.

Time is your resource. Not your ruler.

And when you treat it like the currency it is—with boundaries, discernment, and care—you begin to move through your day with intention, not just momentum.

You begin to see that reclaiming your time isn't selfish—it's survival. It's sovereignty.

You are not behind. You are arriving.

Section Four
Putting On Your Mask Daily

This isn't the end. It's the beginning of choosing you.

The first time I flew alone, I remembered the safety instructions like a mantra: *In the event of a loss of cabin pressure, secure your own oxygen mask before assisting others.*

It made sense in theory. But it wasn't how I was living. At all. Full stop.

For years, I tried to help everyone else breathe while gasping for air myself. I said yes to things that drained me. I overcommitted, overfunctioned, and overexplained. I didn't realize I was becoming resentful—resuntful not because I didn't want to be generous, but because I literally had nothing left to give physically, emotionally, or financially.

It took hitting emotional and physical walls before I realized this truth: self-care is not selfish. It's how I stay alive. Not just physically—but emotionally, mentally, and spiritually.

That's what this section is about.

Section 4 is where theory becomes rhythm. It's where permission becomes practice. Where your healing becomes part of your daily breath and not something you wait until vacation or burnout to allow.

This section is your reminder that:

- You don't have to earn care.

- You don't need a breakdown to justify a break.

- You are allowed to choose yourself—every single day.

Because this isn't about becoming someone new. It's about coming home to yourself, over and over again.

Let's begin.

Chapter Eighteen
Marking your Milestones

"When you say yes to others, make sure you are not saying no to yourself." – Paulo Coehlo

---

I was sitting on the floor of my closet when I realized how much I had been carrying. The laundry was clean but unfolded and scattered everywhere. My phone was constantly buzzing with unanswered messages and social media notifications. My body was aching in ways I didn't even have names for. I had been holding my breath both metaphorically and literally—for months. And that evening, in the quiet between tasks I could no longer pretend to manage, I just...exhaled.

Not a dramatic movie exhale. Not a breakdown. Just a soft, surrendered breath.

Because for once, I had nothing left to perform.

That's when it hit me: I didn't want to live my life waiting for a vacation, a breakdown, or a permission slip. I wanted to live it, not survive it. That realization felt less like fireworks and more like a cracked window letting in fresh air, and, boy, did I need it desperately.

If you're reading this, maybe you've had a moment like that too.

Maybe your version wasn't a closet. Maybe it was the car. Or the bathroom. Or in the middle of a Zoom call you smiled your way through while emotionally dissociating. Wherever it was, what matters is, you made it here. To this moment.

And I want to pause and acknowledge that.

You Did Something Brave

You didn't just read a book.

You confronted some hard truths about your energy, your boundaries, your mindset, and your needs.

You allowed yourself to question the lie that said you have to be constantly productive to be worthy.

You made space to reflect, not just react. You allowed yourself to feel tired and still believe you're worthy of care.

That's not small. That's incredibly courageous.

Healing is a radical act in a world that literally profits off and glorifies your burnout. Choosing yourself is resistance in a culture that teaches you to disappear inside other people's expectations. Actually showing up for your healing is one of the most powerful things you can do.

Even if you still feel like a mess. Even if nothing in your external world has changed yet.

You Were Never Broken—You Were Overburdened

Let's be clear about something: You were never the problem.

The systems, expectations, and beliefs that taught you to overfunction, overgive, and overlook yourself—those were the problem. Not you.

You didn't need to be fixed. You needed to be seen. To be heard. To be given the permission (and language) to name what's been hurting.

You're not selfish for wanting more rest. You're not lazy for needing to unplug.

You're not weak for feeling overwhelmed.

You're human! And being human means you are allowed to need things. Space. Rest. Connection. Silence. A slower pace. Permission to say NO. A gentle reminder that NO is a full sentence.

Healing Isn't Linear. But It's Worth It.

Some days, you'll feel clear. Capable. Grounded.

Other days, you'll forget everything you've read and feel like you're starting from scratch.

That's okay.

Progress isn't always a straight line. Sometimes it looks like pausing. Sometimes it looks like spiraling back into old patterns, but this time, actively noticing the signs sooner. Choosing differently. Recovering faster.

This isn't about perfection. It's about presence and permission to return to yourself, again and again and again.

You Are Becoming Your Own Safe Place

If you've made it this far, it means you're building something new.

A version of yourself who no longer waits to collapse before resting. Who knows that boundaries aren't walls—they're doors to clarity. Who isn't interested in impressing anyone if it means abandoning themselves.

You are becoming the kind of person who breathes deeper, listens to their body, and reclaims their time. You are refusing to apologize for protecting your peace.

That version of you already exists. This book just helped you see yourself more clearly.

Reflection Prompts

Take a few moments to sit with the following questions:

1. What surprised me about my burnout story? What truths did I uncover?

2. What new boundary, mindset, or rhythm do I want to take with me into the next season?

3. How do I want to remind myself—daily—that I deserve care, without guilt or delay?

4. When I look at my life today, what's one small sign that I've grown?

Write freely. Be honest. Let this be your moment to witness yourself.

Final Thoughts – Oxygen Mask Moment

Put your hand on your chest.

Take a breath.

You don't need to rush to the next thing.

You've done enough.

This is your **oxygen mask moment**:

The moment you stop waiting to be worthy.

The moment you stop trying to earn your rest.

The moment you remember you already have permission.

You are allowed to breathe.

You are allowed to do less.

You are allowed to come back to yourself.

This book might be ending—but your journey back to yourself is just beginning.

Every time you choose yourself, it counts, even if no one sees it but you.

You don't have to collapse to deserve care.

You don't have to prove your exhaustion to earn rest.

You can put your oxygen mask on—every single day.

And that, love, is enough.

Chapter Nineteen
The Oxygen Mask is a Mindset, Not a Moment

"Almost everything will work again if you unplug it for a few minutes, including you." – Anne Lamott

---

The Day I Forgot My Own Advice

I was running late. Again.

My alarm had been snoozed too many times, and the day already felt like it was getting away from me. There were emails I hadn't answered, texts sitting unread, groceries that hadn't been picked up, and a calendar full from morning to night.

I threw on a clean-enough sweater, grabbed a cup of tea, and stepped over a pile of clutter that had taken up permanent residence on my floor, which I was trying desperately to ignore.

My phone went off as I got into the car. It was a client needing something. Another notification from my group chat lighting up with plans I didn't have the capacity for—but would probably say yes to anyway.

And in that moment—between the buzzes, the rushing, and the guilt of feeling behind—I realized something. I had once again forgotten to put on my own oxygen mask.

I hadn't meditated or prayed. I hadn't eaten since the day before. I hadn't even taken a deep breath. I was on auto-pilot. I was back in survival mode, trying to be everything for everyone, without being anything for myself.

Even after writing this book, even after learning what I've learned, I still forgot.

And that's the point of this chapter.

A Mindset, Not a Moment

The oxygen mask metaphor is powerful for a reason. It reminds us of something deeply counterintuitive for those of us who've been taught to give, fix, serve, and perform:

You must care for yourself first.

Not only for others. Not just so you can keep going. But because you matter. You are not a tool for someone else's well-being. You are a whole human being with your own needs, limits, and aspirations.

And yet, the oxygen mask isn't a one-time act.

It's not something you "check off" and move on from. It's a mindset, a practice of returning to yourself over and over again, especially when it's hard and especially when you forget.

Self-care is not about perfection. It's about remembering and returning to you.

Why We Forget

Let's be honest: Choosing ourselves isn't always easy.

Even now, I still sometimes feel guilty when I say no. I still feel behind when I rest. I still battle the deeply ingrained voice that says, you're only valuable and have worth when you're producing.

But here's what I've learned:

Forgetting doesn't mean failing. It just means you're human, and humans (especially ones healing from burnout, overfunctioning, and self-abandonment) need reminders. We need anchors. We need gentle ways to come back home to ourselves.

The Mask Is a Daily Return

Putting your oxygen mask on isn't about becoming perfect at boundaries or suddenly becoming a monk in the mountains.

It's about small, quiet decisions that say: I choose me. Even if just for this breath. This moment. This hour.

It's saying:

- I'm allowed to sit down before the house is clean.

- I'm allowed to say no without guilt.

- I'm allowed not to answer that text right now.

- I'm allowed to rest, even when I'm not at my limit yet.

It's choosing to listen when your body whispers, instead of waiting until it screams.

It's pausing for a deep breath before replying to the email that made your shoulders tense up.

It's canceling the plan because you're not in the space to socialize—and knowing that doesn't make you flaky; it makes you honest.

The Mask Is Not a Luxury. It's a Lifeline.

Some people will still try to tell you that putting yourself first is selfish. Some systems will reward you more when you abandon your own needs. Some habits will whisper that you should "just push through."

But you know better now.

You know that a version of you exists that doesn't need to break to earn a break.

You know that your peace is precious and you can protect it.

You know that rest is a right, not a reward.

You know that your value isn't in how much you give, but in the fact that you exist. And even when you forget, this mindset will still be here. Waiting for you to return.

Self-Compassion Over Perfection

Some days you'll forget to breathe deeply.

Some days you'll scroll instead of stretch.

Some days you'll say yes when you actually meant no.

Let that be okay.

Don't turn self-care into another performance.

Don't turn boundaries into a battleground.

Don't turn rest into a reward you have to earn.

Instead, let your oxygen mask be a moment of grace:

- A deep breath.
- A canceled meeting.
- A pause between tasks.
- A kind word to yourself.

That's the practice. That's the mindset.

That's the oxygen mask.

Reflection Prompts

Let this be a space to return to your center—no judgment, just curiosity:

1. What does it *actually* look like when I forget to put my oxygen mask on?

2. What helps me return to myself without shame or blame?

3. What's one micro-decision I can make this week that reinforces my worth?

4. How can I create a gentle routine or cue that helps me remember to breathe?

Final Thoughts – Oxygen Mask Moment

Let's exhale together.

You've made it to the final chapter, but this is not the end.

This is the beginning of a new way of being—one that isn't rushed, reactive, or rooted in guilt.

This is your **oxygen mask mindset**.

It's not about having it all together. It's about giving yourself permission to start again, as many times as you need to.

Every day, you'll be given countless chances to choose yourself. Some days you will. Some days you won't. Both are okay.

The point is to remember that you are allowed to come back—again and again and again.

Because when you put your oxygen mask on first:

- You breathe clearer.

- You love deeper.

- You live softer.

And that, my friend, is more than enough.

Chapter Twenty
What Burnout Taught Us
(And the Permission to Choose
Differently)

"And the day came when the risk to remain tight in a bud was more painful than the risk it took to blossom." – Anaïs Nin

---

I used to believe burnout was the price of a meaningful life.

That exhaustion meant I was doing something important. That the constant pressure in my chest, the dread on Sunday nights, the tension in my shoulders, and the tears I'd cry quietly while brushing my teeth were all signs of ambition, commitment, even strength. That if I just made it through this week, or the next month, or this job, or this season, then I could finally rest.

But that rest never came.

What did come was the slow, creeping realization that my body was shutting down long before I gave myself permission to.

My burnout didn't start with one bad day. It started with the years I spent ignoring myself. It was death by a thousand self-abandonments: the skipped meals, the "yes" when I meant "no," the unread texts from friends I was too depleted to respond to, the quiet resentment I felt as I poured from an empty cup, again and again.

Burnout taught me a lot. But maybe the biggest lesson was this:

You can't abandon yourself and call it a life.

This realization didn't mark the end of burnout. It marked the beginning of the **reckoning**.

The beginning of asking different questions.

Of telling the truth about what I could no longer carry.

Of unlearning everything I was taught about worth and productivity.

And that's what this chapter is: A reckoning. A remembrance. A **permission slip** to live differently.

Burnout Wasn't Your Fault

Let's start here—because shame has no place in healing:

Burnout is not a personal failure.

You didn't burn out because you're weak or lazy or dramatic. You burned out because you are human in a system that glorifies and promotes pushing ourselves beyond the brink as a win.

We are taught to:

- Glorify exhaustion

- Apologize for rest

- Hustle for our value

- Numb instead of feel

- Help others while ignoring our own needs

But here's what burnout teaches if we're brave enough to listen:

Burnout is not a flaw in your character. It's like a flashing neon sign that says:

You've been overextending yourself for too long and it's no longer sustainable. So STOP IT!

It's not asking you to do more. It's begging you to do differently.

What Burnout Taught Us

Across the pages of this book, and maybe across the pages of your life, you've started to see a new truth emerging. One that doesn't demand perfection but invites compassion.

Let's take a moment to name those truths, so you can carry them forward:

Burnout is a signal—not a sentence.

Burnout isn't the end; it's the invitation. To pause. To breathe. To come back to yourself.

You don't need to rebuild your old life. You need to re-imagine a new one.

Self-care is survival.

You've heard the phrase so many times it almost feels cliché. But let's say it in a new way:

Self-care isn't a bubble bath. It's boundaries. It's bravery. It's belonging to yourself.

Self-care is noticing what you need, and choosing not to ignore it.

It's stepping away from what drains you and stepping toward what restores you.

Time is a boundary.

Time isn't just something you manage; it's something you protect.

And you don't owe every minute of your day to others.

- You're allowed to rest before you're depleted.
- You're allowed to do nothing without explaining.
- You're allowed to walk away from urgency culture.

Time is a form of self-respect.

And you don't have to earn the right to use it for yourself.

Rest is resistance.

Resting in a world that rewards burnout? That's not weakness. That's rebellion.

Every time you choose to stop, to breathe, to soften instead of push, you're refusing to let systems of overwork dictate your worth.

You're saying, "I exist outside of hustle."

You're saying, "I deserve care."

You're saying, "I choose me."

You Have Nothing to Prove

If this book has done anything, I hope it reminded you of one deep truth:

You don't need to earn your right to exist.

You don't need to "do more" to be lovable.

You don't need to constantly explain your needs to be respected.

You don't need to be broken down before you're allowed to rest.

You get to choose yourself, not because you're falling apart, but because you are finally coming back together.

Your Permission Slip (Write It, Own It)

Let's make it official. Grab a pen. Open your Notes app. Say it out loud. Whatever feels right for you.

But write this like a promise you're making to the person who needs your love most—*you*.

I give myself permission to:

Say no without guilt.

- Rest without apology.

- Take up space.

- Care for myself even when others don't understand.

- Let things be messy.

- Pause before I respond.

- Cry without shame.

- Ask for help.

- Set boundaries that feel like freedom.

- Be proud of progress others can't see.

- Return to myself whenever I forget.

- Begin again, as many times as it takes.

- Choose myself—every. single. time.

Now add your own:

- I give myself permission to: _____
- I give myself permission to: _____

This is not a wishlist. It's a declaration.

Reflection Prompts

Take a breath. Grab your journal, or simply think through these with honesty and curiosity:

1. What is one belief about rest, worth, or self-care that I'm ready to unlearn?

2. What permission do I most need to give myself today?

3. What would it look like if I showed up for myself the way I show up for everyone else?

4. When I imagine a life in which I am deeply cared for—what does that feel like?

5. What is one boundary I can set this week to honor my well-being?

Final Thought – Oxygen Mask Moment

You have nothing to lose by choosing yourself. And everything to gain: peace, clarity, presence, joy, ease.

There will still be hard days. You'll still forget sometimes. You might even slip into old patterns. That's okay. The difference is, now, you'll know how to return. And you'll know that you're allowed to.

Breathe deep.

Choose yourself.

Put your oxygen mask on.

And live.

Chapter Twenty-One
But What Happens When You're Neuro-Spicy?

I found out I had ADHD and anxiety last year.

And I don't mean I just suspected it. I mean a full-on, official diagnosis, with receipts, checklists, and the overwhelming realization that the way my brain has always worked... had a name. Actually, two names.

For years, I had been walking around as a master of spotting ADHD in others. I could see the signs, the struggles, the brilliance. I mean, I "diagnosed" one of my twin sons at 6 months old and everyone told me I was crazy. I could coach someone through an anxiety spiral with one hand while juggling a to-do list with the other. But somehow, I didn't see it in myself. I thought I was just... chaotic. Or inconsistent. I thought I was incredible at multi-tasking. Or "too much on some days and too quiet on others."

Turns out, I'm Neuro-Spicy. And honestly? That revelation felt like opening a window I didn't know was closed. The fresh air hit, and suddenly, things made sense. The constant mental tabs open. The hyperfocus that made me forget to eat. The sensory overload that showed up in loud cafes or cluttered inboxes. The guilt over needing more rest than others. The struggle with time wasn't just about poor planning—it was about time blindness.

And while the diagnosis gave me language and clarity, it also gave me permission.

Permission to stop trying to fix something that was never actually broken.

Permission to adapt the Oxygen Mask Mindset and C.A.R.E. Tool not just for busy people or burnt-out folks- but for me. For Neurospicy Calissa.

For "I-need-ten-reminders-and-a-playlist-to-clean-the-kitchen" me. For "my emotions-come-in-technicolor" me. For "I'll-do-it-in-five-minutes-unless-I-forget-I-exist" me.

So if you're reading this and thinking, "Okay but what happens when my brain doesn't work like everyone else's?" Well this chapter is for you.

Let's talk about what self-care looks like when you're not only burnt out, but wired differently from the jump.

The Oxygen Mask Mindset for the Neuro-spicy

Here's the truth: every single tool in this book still applies. But the way you use them might have to bend to fit the way your brain works. And that's not a weakness. That's wisdom.

When you're neurodivergent, self-care isn't just about taking breaks or setting boundaries. It's about designing your life in a way that actually works for your brain instead of constantly working against it.

You're not lazy. You're managing executive function overload.

You're not flaky. You're living in a world built for neurotypical timing.

You're not too sensitive. You're carrying a finely tuned emotional radar.

You're not too much. You've just never been given enough space to stretch.

So let's reintroduce the **C.A.R.E. Tool**—your blueprint for sustainable care—but now through the lens of being Neuro-spicy.

C.A.R.E. for the Neurodivergent Nervous System

Clarity: Clear ≠ Rigid

You may need to externalize clarity. That means writing it down, color-coding it, saying it out loud, or using alarms with funny names like "Drink water, you dehydrated sunflower."

Clarity might come from visual timers, sticky notes, or breaking one task into three smaller ones. It's not about being perfect. It's about creating a reality where you can see what's next, and trust yourself to do it.

Pro tip: Clarity for a neurodivergent brain often means simplifying the overwhelm. Start with:

- "What actually needs to happen today?"

- "What will happen if I don't do this right now?"

- "Is this urgent, or just noisy?"

Activity: Movement = Medicine

Sometimes the body needs to move before the brain can focus. Pacing while on the phone, stretching in between Zoom calls, or doing a five-minute "vibe reset" dance party might be how you regulate.

If you struggle to "start" things, give yourself a physical cue. That might look like putting on a hoodie to signal focus time, or lighting a candle when it's time to journal.

Restlessness doesn't mean you're failing. It means your body is speaking. Listen.

Resilience: Emotionally Flexible, Not Emotionless

Neuro-spicy folks often feel more. That's not a flaw; it's a feature. You may carry deep empathy, sensitivity to injustice, or a radar for emotional undercurrents in a room.

But that also means overstimulation, decision fatigue, and emotional exhaustion can hit faster. Resilience, for you, is about creating space for your emotions without drowning in them.

Let yourself cry in the car. Scream into a pillow. Voice note your feelings. Name your needs. Ask for help, even if it feels uncomfortable.

And remember: rest is emotional repair. Not a reward.

Engagement: Connection Your Way

You don't have to be the life of the party. You don't have to respond to every text in five minutes. Your version of social self-care might be one meaningful conversation a week. Or a group chat with friends who understand that "I love you" sometimes sounds like "I need to disappear for two days."

Engagement is not about *more people*—it's about safe *people*.

Engagement might also mean advocating for accommodations, being honest about your capacity, or finding online communities where you feel less alone.

And on the Days You Forget...

Because you will. Because I do often.

There will be days when you fall into doom scrolling, cancel all your plans, or say yes when you meant no.

There will be days when your brain feels like too much, and you feel like not enough.

There will be moments when you are so overstimulated and overwhelmed that your recharge looks like lying in bed all day, watching Netflix, and ordering takeout.

On those days, come back to your tools. Come back to your breath. Come back to your *truth*:

You are not broken. You are beautifully built different.

You do not need to earn your right to care.

You get to exist in a way that works for you, and that is a revolution.

Reflection Prompts

- When did I first notice I felt "different," and what did I believe about myself at the time?

- What strategies have helped me feel more grounded, focused, or seen in my daily life?

- Where am I still trying to "force" myself into systems that don't serve me?

- What might self-care look like if I honored the way my brain and body actually function?

Final Thought – Oxygen Mask Moment

"Your brain isn't a burden. It's a blueprint for your brilliance." Unknown

You don't have to fit someone else's version of productivity to be worthy.

You don't need to shrink or contort to be accepted.

You deserve a life that feels good to live in and one that honors your unique wiring, rhythms, and magic.

The Oxygen Mask Mindset isn't a one-size-fits-all strategy. It's a daily invitation to choose yourself in the way that only *you* can. Loudly, quietly, creatively, awkwardly—whatever works.

Because when you put your mask on first, your way?

You don't just survive. You shine.

Chapter Twenty-Two
The Oxygen Mask Mindset—An Invitation to Keep Going

"When you recover or discover something that nourishes your soul and brings joy, care enough about yourself to make room for it in your life." – Jean Shinoda Bolen

---

Let me be blunt: You made it. Not just to the end of this book, but to the beginning of something far more important.

You didn't just read these pages. You chose yourself, one truth-telling paragraph at a time. You paused. You reflected. You asked hard questions and sat with honest answers. And whether you journaled every prompt or skimmed through with a side-eye and a snack, you showed up. YOU did that, and it matters.

It matters because here's the thing they don't always tell you in self-help books: Choosing yourself doesn't require a total life overhaul. It requires daily, intentional acts of remembering that you matter. Even if you fall back into old habits. Try again. And again. And Again. Until it becomes a habit.

Let me say that again for the perfectionists in the back: You don't need to fix yourself. You just need to come home to yourself. Again and again.

Let's Be Real: Life Will Get Loud Again

This isn't the part where I tell you everything will now be easy and stress-free because you read this book. (I mean, I wish. But I'm not a magician. I'm a writer.)

Life will get loud again.

The calendar will fill. The emails will pile up. The people-pleasing voice will creep back in, whispering that maybe you should say yes, that maybe you should be doing more, and that resting is selfish.

But now? Now you have a different voice inside you too.

One that says:

Pause. You don't need to prove anything. You're allowed to breathe.

This voice is your oxygen mask mindset. Keep it close. It's your anchor when the waves get high again.

Remember the C.A.R.E. Tool?

Oh yes, she's back.

The C.A.R.E. Tool isn't just a cute acronym. It's your burnout recovery compass. Let's bring her back home, one last time:

- **C – Clarity**: You now know what matters. You've defined your values, named your limits, and un-learned the idea that your worth is tied to your productivity.

- **A – Activity**: You've explored what fills you up and what drains you. You've learned how to choose nourishing over numbing.

- **R – Resilience**: You've been reminded that healing isn't about perfection. It's about coming back to yourself, even when you wander. Especially when you wander.

- **E – Engagement**: You've reconnected with what lights you up and gives your life meaning. You've practiced showing up fully, not just functionally.

If all you take from this book is to pause for a deep breath and ask, "What do I need right now?" then you're already practicing the C.A.R.E. Tool.

And that, my friend, is everything.

Let's Drop Some Truth Bombs

Because I know you're here for the realness:

- Burnout steals more than your energy; it steals your joy, your creativity, your presence.

- Rest is not earned. It's required.

- You are allowed to set boundaries without giving a TED Talk about it.

- If they only love the version of you that never says no, they don't love you; they love your compliance.

- Choosing yourself may disappoint others. That's okay. You weren't put on this earth to keep everyone else comfortable.

And if no one has told you lately: You don't have to hold your breath to keep the peace. You deserve to exhale. Fully.

Next Steps (Because This Isn't Goodbye)

This book isn't a conclusion. It's your invitation to keep going. To live this mindset. To return to yourself when you drift.

Here are a few things to keep your oxygen mask mindset alive:

Revisit these pages when life gets messy. Come back to the tools, the truths, the reminders. Dog-ear your favorite chapters. Highlight the permission slips.

Create your own Oxygen Mask Moments. These are small rituals you can return to daily: a 5-minute stretch, a quiet cup of tea, journaling before bed, saying "no" and meaning it.

Join a community. Healing is powerful, but it's exponential when done in connection. Whether it's a group built around this message or one you create for yourself, don't do this alone.

Keep journaling. Let this book be the first of many conversations you have with yourself.

Final Thought – Oxygen Mask Moment

You've read every chapter. You've paused. Reflected. You've let some things go, and maybe picked a few new things up. You've remembered how to come home to yourself.

So here's your final truth:

> **You don't have to prove your worth by burning out.**
> **You don't have to stay silent to stay safe.**
> **You don't have to wait for permission**
> **to put yourself first.**

You. Deserve. To. Breathe.

Not just survive. But breathe—deeply, wildly, and without apology.

This is your Oxygen Mask Mindset.

Keep it close.

Return to it often.

You're worth it.

Author's Note

When I came up with the concept and started writing *The Oxygen Mask Mindset*, I wasn't just trying to write a book.

I was trying to breathe.

I was trying to find language for the exhaustion I couldn't explain. I was trying to piece together the tiny moments of clarity that came between burnout cycles. I was trying to understand how someone who "knew better" could still struggle so deeply with choosing themselves consistently.

And maybe, like you, I was tired of being told that self-care was bubble baths, vacations, and gratitude journals—because the stress was still there when I returned. I discovered that what I really needed was boundaries, space, and the permission to stop performing strength while silently falling apart.

This book became what I needed: a reminder, a reclamation, a roadmap. It became a declaration that healing doesn't require perfection. That choosing yourself isn't selfish—it's a form of resistance in a world that glorifies our exhaustion and benefits when we abandon ourselves.

Writing this wasn't always graceful. Sometimes I had to step away. Honestly, often. Sometimes I cried mid-sentence. Sometimes I laughed out loud at my own sass (I am actually hilarious at times). Sometimes I questioned whether I was allowed to say some of the things I did. But I kept going, because I believed, deeply, that someone out there needed to hear it in this exact way.

Maybe that someone is you.

If you've made it this far, let me say what I wish someone had said to me:

I'm so proud of you. Honestly.

Not because you finished the book. But because you showed up. You listened inward. You paused, reflected, and asked hard questions. You faced truths you maybe hadn't dared to name before. You remembered, maybe for the first time in a long time, that your well-being matters.

You matter.

And I hope *The Oxygen Mask Mindset* becomes something you return to. Not because it holds every answer, but because it opens up the conversation and holds space for you to ask better questions. I hope the C.A.R.E. Tool lives in your back pocket. I hope you write your own permission slips. I hope you create rituals and rhythms that remind you of who you are.

And I hope you breathe—deeply, freely, and unapologetically.

This isn't the end. This is the beginning of choosing you. Again. And again. And again.

Thank you for going on this journey with me.

With gratitude and bold love,

Calissa Ngozi

P.S. If you're ever wondering if you're allowed to slow down, take up space, or just exist exactly as you are, consider this your forever permission slip.

About the Author

Calissa Ngozi is a mental health educator, award-winning speaker, and TV and media guest contributor on nationally syndicated television and radio programming. She is also a Child & Youth Care Professor and business owner based in Ontario, Canada.

Creator of the **Oxygen Mask Mindset™**, Calissa champions radical self-care, boundary-setting, and emotional well-being. Her frameworks and real-talk approach have energized corporate teams, caregivers, educators, parents, and leadership groups across Canada and beyond.

Renowned for her humor, deep empathy, and bold authenticity, Calissa blends personal stories—from fostering success at dawn to burnout breakdowns at midnight—with practical strategies that can be used in boardrooms, bedrooms, and kitchen tables alike.

On top of her professional journey, she's a mom to twin boys, avid traveler, self-declared foodie, and unapologetic nap lover who loves Coldplay. She brings that grounded energy to every stage, workshop, and page she writes.

Calissa lives by the belief that **self-care isn't selfish—it's necessary**. She created **The Oxygen Mask Mindset ™** to help people reclaim their energy so they can show up fully for others and themselves. When she's not teaching, speaking, or running her mental health business, she's happily doing life alongside her community, and she welcomes you to join in the journey.

To connect with Calissa to speak at your event, facilitate a workshop, and more, you can follow her on her Instagram at @calissangozi or her website www.calissangozi.com

thank you

Thank you for reading my book!

Dear Reader,

You made it!!!

Thank you for giving me the space to share my personal stories and examples, my framework, strategies, and empowerments with you.

I hope this book gave you the space to share your story, the opportunity to rest and reflect, and the confidence to reclaim your energy, embrace self-care and set your boundaries with no regrets. It means more than I can describe that we did this together.

Now, if I could ask a quick favour: if you enjoyed the book, would you mind leaving a positive review on Amazon or Goodreads? It would truly make my day, and it's one of the best ways to help others find this book and make my dream a reality! Your review might just be the encouragement someone else needs to empower them to put themselves first and say NO to burnout!

With love,

Calissa Ngozi

MY GIFT TO YOU

I am so glad you're here!

As my Gift to you, get FREE Access to
The Oxygen Mask Mindset bonus content
by scanning the QR Code below or visiting

www.CalissaNgozi.com/books

www.ingramcontent.com/pod-product-compliance
Lightning Source LLC
Chambersburg PA
CBHW070109030426
42335CB00016B/2075